# SUPPORTING SLCN IN CHILDREN WITH ASD IN THE EARLY YEARS

With growing numbers of children with autism spectrum disorder (ASD) being diagnosed in the early years, it is becoming increasingly important for education and health professionals to understand ASD and to implement supportive strategies as part of the everyday curriculum and routine. This book serves as an essential tool kit for anyone working with young children with ASD and speech, language, and communication needs (SLCN). Filled with practical and up-to-date tips, advice, and guidance, it shifts the responsibility of change from the child onto the caregiver, asking the question: what can we do to support the child?

Key features of this book include the following:

- An introduction to ASD

- Detailed case studies illustrating the varied impacts ASD can have on the life of a child

- Practical activities and resources, including planning sheets and activity suggestions

- Easy-to-follow chapters focussing on the classroom environment, communication, social interaction, play, and behaviour

Comprehensive, practical, and evidence based, this manual is essential reading for anyone working with children experiencing social communication difficulties and ASD in an early years setting.

**Jennifer Warwick** trained as a speech and language therapist in 2003; she has wide-ranging experience with children and young people with ASD and other complex communication needs across both the National Health Service (NHS) and charitable sector and in independent practice (www.londoncommunicationclinic.com). Jennifer is currently undertaking a part-time PhD at City University of London and is committed to research and best practice. She is a joint author of the Early Sociocognitive Battery (ESB) and trains speech therapists to use the assessment tool. Jennifer designs and runs training programmes for parents and professionals to support their knowledge in developing communication skills. In addition to clinical work she has managed and supervised a team of therapists and continues to provide clinical supervision and training to others. She is an advisor for ASD and social communication and research champion for the Royal College of Speech and Language Therapists (RCSLT). Jennifer is passionate about improving outcomes in the children and young people she works with.

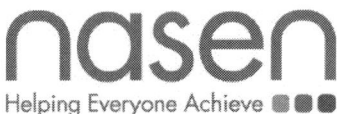

**nasen** is a professional membership association that supports all those who work with or care for children and young people with special and additional educational needs. Members include teachers, teaching assistants, support workers, other educationalists, students, and parents.

**nasen** supports its members through policy documents, journals, its magazine *Special*, publications, professional development courses, regional networks, and newsletters. Its website contains more current information, such as responses to government consultations. **nasen's** published documents are held in very high regard both in the UK and internationally.

Other titles published in association with the National Association for Special Educational Needs (nasen):

*Supporting Children with Cerebral Palsy, 2ed*
Rob Grayson, Jillian Wing, Hannah Tusiine, Graeme Oxtoby, and Elizabeth Morling
2017/pb: 978-1-138-18742-9

*More Trouble with Maths: A Teacher's Complete Guide to Identifying and Diagnosing Mathematical Difficulties, 2ed*
Steve Chinn
2016/pb: 978-1-138-18750-4

*Supporting Children with Dyslexia, 2ed*
Hilary Bohl and Sue Hoult
2016/pb: 978-1-138-18561-6

*Dyslexia and Early Childhood*
Barbara Pavey
2016/pb: 978-0-415-73652-7

*The SENCO Survival Guide, 2ed*
Sylvia Edwards
2016/pb: 978-1-138-93126-8

*Supporting Children with Sensory Impairment*
Gill Blairmires, Cath Coupland, Tracey Galbraith, Elizabeth Morling, Jon Parker, Annette Parr, Fiona Simpson, and Paul Thornton
2016/pb: 978-1-138-91919-8

For a full list of titles see: www.routledge.com/nasen-spotlight/book-series/FULNASEN

# SUPPORTING SLCN IN CHILDREN WITH ASD IN THE EARLY YEARS

## A PRACTICAL RESOURCE FOR PROFESSIONALS

Jennifer Warwick

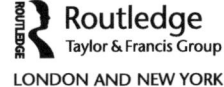

Routledge
Taylor & Francis Group
LONDON AND NEW YORK

First published 2020
by Routledge
2 Park Square, Milton Park, Abingdon, Oxon OX14 4RN

and by Routledge
52 Vanderbilt Avenue, New York, NY 10017

*Routledge is an imprint of the Taylor & Francis Group, an informa business*

© 2020 Jennifer Warwick

The right of Jennifer Warwick to be identified as author of this work has been asserted by her in accordance with sections 77 and 78 of the Copyright, Designs and Patents Act 1988.

All rights reserved. The purchase of this copyright material confers the right on the purchasing institution to photocopy pages which bear the photocopy icon and copyright line at the bottom of the page. No other part of this publication may be reproduced, stored in a retrieval system, or transmitted in any form or by any means, electronic, mechanical, photocopying, recording or otherwise, without prior permission in writing from the publisher.

*Trademark notice*: Product or corporate names may be trademarks or registered trademarks, and are used only for identification and explanation without intent to infringe.

*British Library Cataloguing-in-Publication Data*
A catalogue record for this book is available from the British Library

*Library of Congress Cataloging-in-Publication Data*
A catalog record for this book has been requested

ISBN: 978-1-138-36948-1 (hbk)
ISBN: 978-1-138-36950-4 (pbk)
ISBN: 978-0-429-42862-3 (ebk)

Typeset in DIN Pro
by Apex CoVantage, LLC

# CONTENTS

**Acknowledgements**   vii

**Introduction to autism spectrum disorder (ASD)**   1

This chapter provides relevant background and theory to help you 'get in the shoes' of children with ASD.

**The early years environment: challenges and opportunities**   42

This chapter discusses the early years environment and provides a range of strategies to help increase understanding in the early years environment through use of visual supports, routines, and structured teaching.

**Communication skills**   81

This chapter considers how communication develops typically and the challenges children with ASD face in terms of communication skills. Strategies are provided to develop and support communication within the early years environment.

**Social interaction**   127

This chapter considers the social interaction challenges that young children with ASD face in the early years and provides a range of positive strategies to enable staff to develop a social connection and facilitate interaction.

**Play skills in the early years**   155

Play is a key part of development that we know can be challenging for children with ASD. In this chapter we consider how we can develop play skills in children with ASD.

# Contents

### Making sense of behaviour — 173
Communication difficulties often present themselves as behaviour that challenges. In this chapter we introduce tools to help make sense of behaviour and strategies to support reducing and preventing behaviour difficulties.

### Next steps — 193

### Appendices — 195
*Appendix One: Understanding ASD quiz* 195
*Appendix Two: Strategy planning* 197
*Appendix Three: Let's create planning sheet* 199
*Appendix Four: Communication profile* 200
*Appendix Five: Interaction planner* 202

# ACKNOWLEDGEMENTS

Thank you to The Hanen Centre and FIRST WORD® Project for giving permission to use their valuable work as part of this resource.

With thanks to Becky, Imogen, and Alice, who have so kindly shared their insights in contributing to this manual.

A huge thank you to my family and especially Alex for everything that he does.

With thanks to my supportive colleagues Leonie Kenny, speech and language therapist, and Dr. Rachael McCarthy, clinical psychologist, for their positivity and encouragement.

Finally a thank you to all the inspirational children, parents, and educators I have met along the way.

# Chapter One
# INTRODUCTION TO AUTISM SPECTRUM DISORDER (ASD)

**Chapter One provides the following:**

- An overview of this manual and how to use it
- An overview of ASD to support your understanding
- Background theory and relevant perspectives
- Sensory processing difficulties, the occupational therapist (OT) perspective
- Case study examples and practical activities
- The child's perspective of ASD
- Introduction to the Information-Gathering Tool
- Introduction to the Skills Profile
- Insight into the process of getting a diagnosis and the parental perspective

## Using this manual

- This manual has been written for people working with children with ASD in the early years environment. The manual will also be useful for parents and carers. You may be a teaching assistant, teacher, SENCO, health-care professional, or student. Regardless of your background I hope you find a wealth of information and practical ideas.

- Whilst I have tried to avoid technical terms and unnecessary theory, it is important to have a background understanding of what ASD is and how this impacts a child. Without this context, it can be hard to understand why a child is presenting a certain way, why you are using a particular approaches, and how then to modify your practise. I urge you to read the theory and take time to digest it.

# Introduction to autism spectrum disorder (ASD)

- There is a lot of information in this manual! It may be that you choose to implement relevant strategies chapter by chapter over a period of time. Effecting change takes time, and introducing new strategies needs time to allow for consistency and for them to become embedded. The manual aims to be a practical resource that you can revisit.

- One of the key parts of this manual is the Skills Profile and Information-Gathering Tool which we introduce to you in Chapter One. These are tools that can be used flexibly in your setting. You can reuse them many times and include them as part of your regular observations you make on a child.

- Each chapter has a range of activity sheets to accompany it. These are practical ideas of how to support a child. They are written in a simple and user-friendly way and are designed to be accessible. They can be copied and included in a child's planning/personal folder and learning journey to make sure that they are accessible.

- Activity sheets can be used for a whole nursery approach or to use one on one with an individual child. The activities can also be used in groups.

The manual uses a series of icons to help the reader break information down:

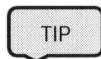 Look for the tip speech bubble for helpful hints and reminders.

 Look for the recap star for helpful summaries of information that has been covered in more detail.

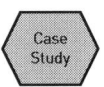 Look for the case study icon for case studies to illustrate examples.

 Look out for the activity icon that you can use individually or as a small group.

## First things first: understand ASD

Understanding the nature of ASD is crucial to being able to effectively support children within the early years environment.

As a parent or educator one of the best things you can do is to **'get into the shoes'** of a child with ASD and see the world from his or her perspective.

Although children with ASD may share the same diagnosis, they will all present differently. The following well-known quote illustrates this perfectly.

*If you have met one person with autism . . . you've met one person with autism.*

Dr. Stephen Shore

# Introduction to autism spectrum disorder (ASD)

Approaching each child that you meet with ASD in an open minded way will help both the child and the parents.

It's no surprise that many ASD organisations and charities have a puzzle as part of their logo. To me this represents ASD well insofar as, like a puzzle, there are many individual parts and factors. Unlike many conditions in which you can have a blood test or scan to give you a diagnosis, ASD requires gathering information over time. As educators, you can help by understanding each piece of the puzzle. Supporting children with ASD can be a bit like completing a puzzle; there are many interlinking parts that need to all fit together.

## What is ASD?

Autism, autism spectrum continuum, Asperger's?

There are many terms used to describe ASD. This can be a little bit confusing.

The *Diagnostic and Statistical Manual of Mental Disorders*, Fifth Edition (DSM-5), published by the American Psychiatric Association (2013), recommended the term 'autism spectrum disorder' as an umbrella term. This effectively replaced other labels for ASD. We use the term ASD throughout this manual. ASD is defined by DSM-5 as 'persistent difficulties with social communication and social interaction' and 'restricted and repetitive patterns of behaviours, activities or interests' that are present from early childhood that 'limit and impair everyday functioning'.

ASD, as its name suggests, covers a broad group of people with a wide and varying range of needs. Whilst everyone with ASD may present differently, to receive a diagnosis of ASD, a person will need to present with persistent difficulties across two key areas: social communication and interaction skills and restricted and repetitive behaviours. This is illustrated in Figure 1.1.

ASD can also be accompanied by varying degrees of learning difficulties, which can impact the child's ability to access the curriculum and engage with learning opportunities. When considering the whole picture, it is important to be aware of any cognitive difficulties that a child may have.

ASD used to be thought of as a condition that affected mostly boys and men. However, there is more and more research indicating that girls with ASD are missed or misdiagnosed. Girls with ASD do present differently, which is important to bear in

# Introduction to autism spectrum disorder (ASD)

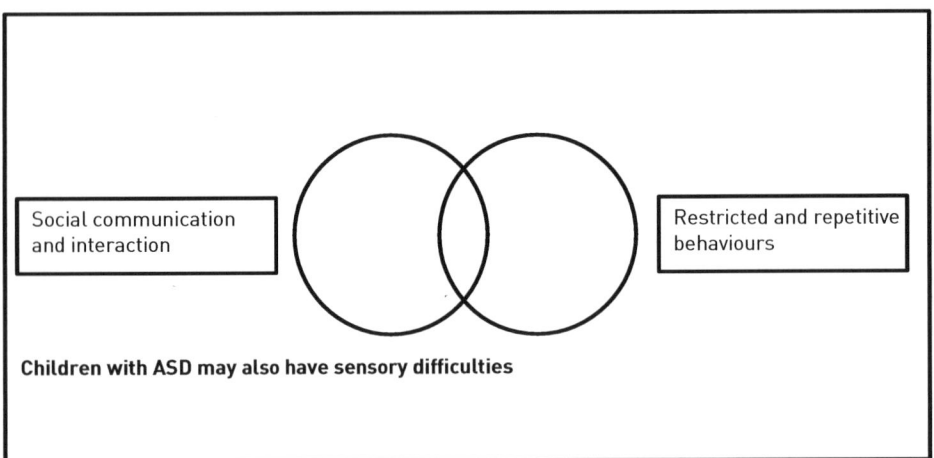

Figure 1.1

mind when you meet children in the early years. We will discuss gender differences in ASD later on in this chapter.

We all have a role in spreading ASD awareness to help the children we work with and their families, so it is important to have as much understanding as possible about the strengths and challenges.

We will now look in more detail at the two key areas associated with a diagnosis of ASD.

Remember not all children with ASD will present the same way, so with certain children in mind, you may identify with some of the characteristics that follow and not with others. Difficulties in some or all of these areas mean that making sense of the social world and those around them can be a real challenge. Children with ASD often require help and support in doing things that for most children come naturally. Symptoms of ASD also change in a child over time depending on other factors in their lives.

## Social communication and interaction difficulties – what you might see?

### *Communication*

- **Difficulties developing communication in a typical way** – Children with ASD struggle to make requests, and it can be difficult for them to 'ask' for items in a typical way. They may not understand that they need to send you a message so will attempt to get something themselves or stand and scream near the item that they want. Even for children who are verbal, requesting can be difficult.

- **Difficulties with expressive language** – Often a first sign of any need may be a lack of typical language development. Children with ASD present with diverse expressive language profiles ranging from children who are completely non-verbal to those who talk articulately about a wide range of subjects. Difficulties with expression are discussed in more detail in Chapter Three.

- **Difficulties with receptive language** – As with expressive language, children with ASD may present with a wide range of needs in terms of their understanding. Some children with ASD may not understand words at all and rely on pictures and symbols whereas others can understand complex verbal information. Difficulties with understanding are discussed in more detail in Chapters Two and Three.

- **Lack of pointing** – At a young age, children with ASD may struggle to point to request and to share interest (pointing to show something interesting to another person).

- **Lack of gestures** – Children who just have speech and language difficulties will try and send you a message using gestures and pointing. Often children with ASD will not do this. Children with ASD may not wave, nod, or shake their heads as other children do. In Chapter Three we talk about typical communication development and highlight the role of gesture use. The 16 gestures by 16 months from the FIRST WORDS PROJECT® in Chapter Three provides a useful overview.

- **Unusual patterns of language, for example, echolalia** (repeated language) – This may be immediately repeating you or delaying; for example, when you say, 'Would you like a drink', the child will say back to you, 'Would you like a drink?'. Children with ASD may also use **repetitive or stereotyped language**, for example, reciting a story or favourite TV programme. This may occur at the correct time, or it may occur at a time that is inappropriate.

- **Difficulties with tone of voice, volume, rate of speech (both using and understanding)** – Sometimes children with ASD will talk in a way that is different from other children and seem unaware of this, for example, talking at an unusual volume or in a different accent. Children with ASD may also find it difficult to pick up on when adults changes their tone to communicate.

# Introduction to autism spectrum disorder (ASD)

- **Difficulties with non-verbal communication** – Children with ASD may struggle to understand and use facial expressions and body proximity in a typical way. This may mean that sometimes they don't get it right, for example, showing a lack of physical boundaries at carpet time by leaning on all the other children. Some children with ASD can show a mismatch in their facial expressions and how they are actually feeling, for example, feeling happy but showing a blank expression. These difficulties with non-verbal communication mean that children with ASD may struggle to understand how you are feeling from your facial expression. Often typically developing children are able to pick up on these more subtle cues and modify their behaviour when an adult shows a particular expression; this is much harder for children with ASD.

- **Difficulties with more abstract and non-literal language** – Children with ASD may find it hard to understand implied meaning, some jokes, and figures of speech.

## *Interaction*

- **Unusual eye contact** – This may be reduced or too intense. Some children with ASD show good eye contact on their terms when they want to but might not look at you when you would usually expect, for example, when you call their names or say, 'Well done, Jack'.

- **Difficulties with joining in with others** – Children with ASD may not be motivated by social interactions in the same way other children are. This can result in a child who doesn't always join others in interaction in a typical way.

- **Difficulties with sharing and taking turns** – This is a difficult skill for all children to develop; however, children with ASD are likely to find this harder than other children.

- **Difficulties with conversation skills** – Starting conversations, maintaining conversations, repairing conversations, as well as having a two-way conversations are all areas of difficulty for children with ASD. Often children with ASD will have a particular topic they find interesting, and due to their difficulties with 'reading other people' and social communication difficulties, they may talk at length about this topic and show a lack of awareness that another person may not be interested in this.

# Introduction to autism spectrum disorder (ASD)

- **Difficulties with understanding how other people think and feel** – Children with ASD have difficulties with theory of mind (discussed later in this chapter), which impacts their ability to think about how other people see the world in a different way to them.

- **Difficulties with understanding and regulating their own emotions** – This is something that can be difficult for all developing children in early years; however, children with ASD struggle to develop these skills. Often not being able to articulate how they are feeling and manage this can result in meltdowns.

## Restricted and repetitive behaviours – what might you see?

- **A particular focus or obsession with a favourite activity** – This may mean an intense interest in only playing with one toy, for example, the train.

- **Restricted range of interests, for example, focussing for long periods on a favourite topic** – This may mean that a child knows a lot about this particular topic, for example, outer space.

- **Difficulties with managing change and a preference for routines** – The social world can be extremely confusing for children with ASD; routines can help children feel safe and secure.

- **Repetitive movements** – You may see hand flapping, spinning, or other mannerisms.

- **Difficulties with pretend or imaginative play** – Children with ASD can find play that involves imagination such as dressing up, role play, or tea parties difficult. These difficulties also impact their ability to use objects in an imaginative way beyond their intended purposes, for example, using a banana for a phone. Some children with ASD will engage in pretend play; however, this can have a slightly learnt element, for example, copied from a book or TV programme.

## Sensory processing difficulties

Children with ASD may also have difficulties with sensory processing. Children without ASD can also have difficulties with sensory processing as well (to make it even more complicated to understand!). An occupational therapist (OT) may work with children with ASD to address sensory processing difficulties.

# Introduction to autism spectrum disorder (ASD)

Sensory processing is quite complex; however, having a simple understanding of sensory processing can help you understand why children may be behaving or responding the way they are to certain situations. It may also help you understand whether a referral to an OT is needed.

We are constantly bombarded with sensory information every second of the day: visual, sound, taste, touch, smell, and movement. There are certain times when people who don't have sensory difficulties can find sensory information overwhelming. Think of a time you have been on a crowded and noisy street or train platform. Depending on the day, your mood or level of tiredness, these situations can be more or less of a problem.

People with sensory processing difficulties struggle to make sense of all this sensory information, which can impact them in their daily activities. In children with ASD who have sensory difficulties, coping with these difficulties can result in increased repetitive behaviours or meltdowns.

For people with ASD their senses can be over or under sensitive. Within the early years environment, you may see children who cover their ears in response to certain noises or who refuse to wear a plastic apron or touch or eat certain textures of food. Bear in mind that these difficulties may be linked to sensory needs.

Try to build up a picture as to what factors may be impacting a child and record on the Information-Gathering Tool.

## Sensory processing – the OT perspective

Nikki Queton, specialist children's occupational therapist, provides an overview to sensory processing.

### *What is sensory processing?*

Sensory processing is the ability to take in, sort out, process, and make use of sensory information from the world around us. It allows us to make an appropriate adaptive response (goal-directed response) to meet the demands of the environment (Biel and Peske, 2009). For higher levels of the brain to work effectively, the lower levels must sort out the information accurately. This sensory information goes to the brain, where it is organised and interpreted. Information about one's own body and the world is gathered from seven senses:

- **Touch (tactile sense)** – There are two types of touch systems located under our skin: the protective touch system responds to light or unexpected touch and alerts our bodies to anything that may be potentially dangerous, for example, touching a sharp object. The discriminative touch system tells you where and what is being touched, for example, findings items in your pocket without looking (Stock Kranowitz, 2005).

- **Movement (vestibular sense)** – The vestibular system is our balance and movement sense. It tells us where our bodies are in relation to gravity and whether we are moving and how fast. The movement receptors, located in the inner ear, are important for body posture and the maintenance of a stable visual field (Stock Kranowitz, 2005).

- **Body posture (proprioception)** – Proprioception is the sense that gives us information regarding the location, movement, and posture of our bodies in physical space. Understanding where our bodies are in space is called body schema. Our body schema is our unconscious map of our bodies, almost like a plan inside our heads that tells us where our different body parts are (Stock Kranowitz, 2005).

- **Sight (vision)** – Vision is one of the most powerful senses. Light rays enter our eyes; these are then transformed to electrical signals which are transmitted via the optic nerve to our brains. It is through this process that we are able to perceive the qualities of the world around us. Visual information such as colour, shape, size, and brightness are all processed.

- **Sound (auditory sense)** – Our auditory sense relates to our ability to hear. Hearing is a complex physiological process where sounds in our environment are funneled into the ear canal; they are transformed into signals which are sent to the brain via the auditory nerve and interpreted as sounds.

- **Smell (olfactory sense)** – Our sense of smell is closely linked to our sense of taste and is reported to be one of the most powerful senses linked to memories and experiences. The olfactory system is responsible for our ability to smell. Our sensory organs perceive molecules in the air and then nerve signals are sent to the brain and processed.

- **Taste (gustatory sense)** – Our gustatory sense relates closely to smell in that they both involve perception of molecules. Our taste buds allow us to recognise the five taste sensations of sweet, sour, bitter, salty and umami; this allows us to perceive flavour.

# Introduction to autism spectrum disorder (ASD)

## Why is sensory processing important?

The integration of sensory input allows children to assess daily situations, formulate an action plan, and produce an action (Stock Kranowitz, 2005), for example, seeing a toy on a shelf and standing on one leg and reaching for it with appropriate strength and grip. Additionally, children enjoy activities which develop sensory processing, for example, running, swinging, jumping, as these activities promote brain development and motor skills.

## Dysfunction in sensory processing

For most children, sensory processing develops in the course of ordinary childhood activities. But for some children, sensory processing does not develop as efficiently as it should. This is known as sensory processing disorder (SPD) or dysfunction in sensory processing. Dysfunction in sensory processing does not mean that the brain is damaged but that the information from the senses is not following and integrating efficiently (Stock Kranowitz, 2005).

When the sensory processing process is disordered, a number of problems in learning, motor skills, and behaviour may be evident and can include the following (Stock Kranowitz, 2005):

- Physical clumsiness and co-ordination difficulties
- Difficulty learning new movements
- Activity level unusually high or low
- Poor body awareness
- Inappropriate (under-reactive, over-reactive, or mixed) response to touch, movements, sights, or sounds
- Social and/or emotional difficulties – distractibility, impulsivity, or limited attention control
- Delays in speech, language, and/or motor skills
- Specific learning difficulties and/or perceptual difficulties
- Poor self-care skills – toileting, feeding, washing, dressing, and grooming
- Poor self-esteem as a result of under achieving

## What can we do to help, using different types of sensory input?

It is important to acknowledge that every child is different and that sensory input may differ from child to child. Children can present with sensory behaviours that are sensory seeking, sensory sensitive and avoiding, and being under responsive to the environment and stimuli. Table 1.1 highlights general sensory strategies that can be both calming and stimulating if conducted differently (Biel and Peske, 2009).

Other strategies can assist depending on the presentation of the behaviours:

- Grading of exposure to activities such as messy play when oversensitivity and avoidance is noted
- Increased sensory input in activities for children who are under responsive and sensory seeking
- Using deep pressure and working against gravity to regulate and prevent overstimulation (sensory seeking and being overstimulated)
- Sensory equipment to provide increased sensory input (climbing equipment, swings, trampoline, or scooter) for children who are sensory seeking and also being under responsive
- Sensory diets (provided by an occupational therapist for a detailed plan of intervention)
- Time (do not rush as rushing can increase anxiety)

Table 1.1 General sensory strategies

| Calming | Stimulating |
| --- | --- |
| Deep pressure | Light touch/tickling |
| Soft lighting | Bright, flashing, or fluorescent lights |
| Rhythmic linear touch, e.g., rocking, deep-pressure stroking | Variable, unpredictable touch |
| Linear rhythmic movement | Unpredictable movement, spinning, rotating – advise not to use this |
| Soft, medium voice | Loud, high-pitched, rapid, unpredictable voice |
| Introducing one thing at a time | Lots of different stimuli |
| Calm, soft, rhythmic music | Loud, irregular beat |

## Introduction to autism spectrum disorder (ASD)

- Warnings and communication strategies
- Visuals and timers

Often attention and focus are concerns for children with sensory processing difficulties as it impacts on their learning. Remember the following:

- We all need to keep ourselves alert.
- All children benefit from movement breaks.
- A short break helps keep our brains alert.

### *Assessing sensory processing*

If a child is suspected of having sensory processing difficulties that affect learning and development, it is recommended that he or she be referred to an OT for further assessment. A sensory diet or further advice will be provided to support home and school with facilitating and developing the child's sensory processing skills.

### *What equipment might be useful?*

- Tactile balls
- Stepping stones
- Mini trampoline
- Therapy ball
- Tunnel
- Move 'n' sit cushion
- Noise-cancelling headphones
- Weighted compression vest

### *How can parents and teachers support sensory processing therapy?*

- **Recognise the problem** – Accept that the behaviours presented by the child are as a result of a real problem and the child is behaving in that manner for a reason.
- **Help the child feel 'all right' about himself or herself** – Facilitating a child's engagement in self-care, school tasks, and play (i.e., breaking a task into small

achievable steps and allowing sufficient time for the child to complete it), along with constant reassurance, will help build up skills, confidence, and self-esteem.

- **Control the environment** – Environmental control means that the sensory stimuli (e.g., lighting, noise level, seating, the structure and level of activities, and sufficient time to complete a task) in the learning and home environment are suitable for the child's processing capacity. The therapist can offer advice on environmental modifications at home and in the classroom.

- **Teach the child to play** – Children with sensory processing difficulties may appear clumsy and tend to avoid games and sensory experiences which they may find challenging. Parents and teachers should encourage children to engage in a variety of activities such as climbing, swimming, swinging, riding bike, making art, taking physical education lessons, and playing with variety of toys which have different sizes and textures.

It is important to remember that when a child experiences difficulties in any of these areas, this can lead to confusion and anxiety, which can in turn be seen as difficult behaviour or meltdowns. By understanding the needs of children with ASD to a greater degree, you can help avoid difficult situations and make their world a much easier place.

## Strengths seen in children with ASD

Children with ASD have many strengths that can be effectively used to help them learn new skills. Using a child's strengths and interests is a great place to start in terms of understanding them and how best to support them, for example, using dinosaurs or the solar system to teach other skills.

**TIP** As a tip, I have been to many planning meetings involving education staff, parents, and professionals that often become lengthy discussions about what a child is unable to do. Starting the meeting with strengths, what is going well, can totally change the tone of the meeting.

I have had the pleasure or working with many wonderful children with ASD and their families, and even with the many challenges children can have, there are also strengths. This list is not exhaustive, but here are some that I have observed.

- Good attention to detail

- Strong interest in activities that are motivating to them – having a strong interest can be helpful to introduce other topics, for example, using dinosaurs to teach colours and numbers

# Introduction to autism spectrum disorder (ASD)

- Visual learning skills
- Good sense of right and wrong
- Good sense of humour
- Motivation to learn

## Understanding the full picture

*Activity* Think about a child that you know who has ASD or possible ASD. Think about their strengths and needs, and group these into social communication and interaction difficulties and restricted and repetitive behaviours. Also note down any possible sensory behaviours.

## What causes ASD?

The exact cause of ASD is not yet known. However, it is believed that both genetic and environmental factors are involved. Research involving twins and siblings has shown that ASD can run in families. ASD can also be associated with other conditions and can co-occur with other diagnoses such as Down syndrome, attention deficit hyperactivity disorder (ADHD), and mental health difficulties.

Whilst the exact causes are not known, we do know that the following things do not cause ASD: vaccines or parenting style. There continues to be a lot of misinformation around the causes of ASD which can be misleading and confusing for parents.

The internet can be a confusing place to navigate when trying to find reliable information about ASD. I would always recommend the following websites for useful resources about ASD:

The National Autistic Society (www.nas.org)

The Autism Education Trust (www.autismeducationtrust.org.uk/)

## Gender differences in ASD

ASD has always been thought of as a predominantly male condition. Although there are more boys diagnosed with ASD, there is increasing research into girls with ASD which indicates that girls are often misdiagnosed, diagnosed later in life, or missed. The impact of this on the individual and her family can be significant. Often girls who end up with a diagnosis of ASD can be overlooked in the early years environment as their difficulties can appear more subtle. Research indicates that the interests of girls with ASD are more similar to typical peers, and they may be socially motivated to fit in. This means that often in an early years setting, it may be difficult to always identify their difficulties. I have worked with children who have received a diagnosis of ASD where the education setting has no concerns at all; girls often cover up or 'mask' their difficulties in an effort to appear more like their peers. The process of this 'masking' can be exhausting, which is why there can be a significant discrepancy with how parents or educators see a child. Often when a child gets home, the exhausting process of 'masking' becomes too much, and the difficulties show themselves as meltdowns.

The experience of women and girls with ASD is fascinating, and there are many books and films available about this.

I had the pleasure of speaking at a parent conference about ASD in girls a few years ago; as part of the presentation I was joined by Imogen and her mum. Imogen has a diagnosis of ASD; I met her as part of her diagnostic assessment. Imogen (who was fifteen at the time of writing) has kindly agreed to share her story, which provides a great insight into female ASD.

Imogen was able to give this talk to a lecture hall full of parents, which is truly impressive.

## ASD in girls – Imogen's perspective

### *This is me*

Hi, my name is Imogen. I am fifteen years old. I have autism ;). My favourite colour is purple, and my favourite shape is a circle.

### *Perception of the world and people before the diagnosis*

Before my diagnosis I had a lot of trouble talking to people my age. I could talk to adults and people who were younger than me quite easily, but I struggled with understanding anybody between the ages of ten and thirty. I found it quite stressful being in situations where I didn't know everybody in the room. I hated holiday play schemes. I preferred to sit by myself and read (or even just stare at a wall) until my mother arrived to pick me up. Of course, adults would think that I was sad and lonely.

# Introduction to autism spectrum disorder (ASD)

They would start asking me questions and getting other children to play with me. It was a nightmare. I didn't exactly blend in either; all the kids wanted to play with the mysterious redhead. I didn't want to be rude, so I gritted my teeth and played their games or followed them for an hour. It was awful.

## *Primary school – obligatory purgatory*

I joined my primary school in year two. I'd been in the same nursery as most of my classmates but had moved away for a few years. Everyone knew me as I had been popular in nursery. However, I didn't remember any of them. Well, I remembered one girl, whom I hated (but we're now best friends). Pretty soon, people started to realise there was something different about me. I ended up with just two friends at school. Everyone else didn't like me because I couldn't conform to their norms. I got beaten up once. I was told that violence would get me in trouble, so I stood still, folded my arms, and allowed the girl to hit and kick me. I didn't think to tell a teacher, but one heard the chants of the older students surrounding me and got the girl to stop. Someone asked why I didn't defend myself. I told them, crying, that I didn't want to get into trouble.

I was absolutely obsessed with cats in primary school. I was a cat every Halloween and had learnt how to imitate a cat in their sounds and body language. People noticed this, and I got called a few different names. One was Tiger Girl. They meant it as an insult. I took it as a compliment. That was until the year sixes surrounded me one day, all making animal noises and laughing. I was extremely disoriented as they pretended to claw at me and hiss. I started to lash out; they found that hilarious. Again, the only reason they stopped was because a teacher turned up and restrained me whilst telling them all to leave. I hated school, but I knew I had to attend, otherwise my mother would get into trouble.

## *Triggers and indicators that have led to diagnosis*

I was in therapy from when I was six until I was thirteen; first it was art therapy, then psychotherapy, then cognitive behavioural therapy (CBT). I was told I had 'social anxiety', which I told people when they realised that I wasn't as committed to the conversation as they were. I wasn't making any progress in therapy, and eventually my last therapist suggested that I might have autism. I was articulate, but I didn't respond to anything.

# Introduction to autism spectrum disorder (ASD)

## *My reaction and perception of the diagnosis (good and bad sides)*

I am happy that I have been diagnosed. I now understand why I'm so different to other people, so I can learn how to communicate like them. It also means that I can ask for and get support from my school and clubs. People are also more understanding and forgiving of my social blunders. I find it easier to make friends because of this; they know that I want them to tell me when I have appeared rude so that I can prevent making the same mistake. It means that they don't hold onto rude things I've said or done. They tell me, I apologise, and they don't hold it against me.

## *Other people's reaction to my diagnosis and their disbelief*

When I told my friends that I had autism, they took it as a fact. I don't think they knew what autism was. One boy in my science class asked me why I was so weird; I told him why. He told me that I wasn't autistic. I explained that I was. He then informed me that I couldn't be autistic because I was too 'self-aware'. I was offended. I asked him what he meant by that because I was pretty sure that one of the parts of being a human was self-awareness. He said that I couldn't be autistic because I had said that I had autism and understood what it meant. I then explained that I knew that I was autistic because a professional had diagnosed me a week prior. Then, he said that I couldn't be autistic because I wasn't like the autistic boy in our year. So I told him to shut up because he didn't know what he was talking about – autism is a spectrum; there can be many differences between two autistic people. However, I was wrong – he informed me that his mother was an educational psychologist, so he must know *all* about autism. I told him where he could put his opinion, and we haven't had a conversation since.

This year, another boy got moved into my science class. He sat on a table with only my friend and myself. He announced, one lesson, that someone on the table had something wrong with her brain, but it wasn't him or my friend. I then explained to him that he was in fact correct, but I was still quite offended that he had felt the need to say that. The boy who sits behind me then said, 'We know, Imogen. You keep on saying that'. I told him that I only ever mentioned my diagnosis when somebody asked or mentioned it. I pointed out that the boy had said that I had a brain disability and that I was only telling him that he was not completely wrong.

# Introduction to autism spectrum disorder (ASD)

When my mother told some of her friends that I had a diagnosis of autism, it was interesting to hear of their reactions. My mother said that they mostly did not react at all, except to pull a face. Others responded with disbelief. 'Not Imogen. She's fine – of course she's not autistic'! My mother said that she thinks they have a 'Rainman' image of autism (male idiot savant) – apparently, a film starring Dustin Hoffman – before my time.

## *Challenges of social interaction*

I often find that people will ask me a question and I'm not sure how to answer. I always seem to be the only person who thinks the question is unclear or has too many answers. For example, if someone gives me a list of numbers and asks, 'What is your favourite number?', I will panic. Do they mean a number on the list? Do they want only real numbers; what about imaginary ones? Is there a character limit on my number? I even wonder how long I'm allowed to think about the answer! I usually prefer to be the fifth or seventh person to answer a question. This gives me a chance to listen to other people's answers and create a mental script. However, quite often, I'm asked first or second, so I give a vague answer. This makes people think that I'm upset with them or not focussed. Of course, I'm focussed – I'm just terrified.

Sometimes, at school, I'll be sitting in my form room reading, and one of the girls in my class will sit down in her designated seat, right next to mine. She'll usually start talking to me, asking questions and talking about herself. I feel rude if I don't nod when she speaks or answer her questions. However, I always keep my eyes firmly fixed on my book. I always think that I'm making it pretty clear that I'm busy and I don't want to talk, but I guess she thinks I'm multitasking. I find it frustrating when this happens because, frankly, when I'm reading I don't care if the person talking to me is on fire and begging for me to pour my bottle of water on her. I will always be more interested in the characters in whichever book I'm reading.

Occasionally, I think I make people uncomfortable. As I struggle with creating body language and verbal language appropriate to the situation (especially if it is informal), I will normally copy those generated by the other people in the group. I normally take care to copy parts of all the people present, so it doesn't look like I'm completely mimicking one person. However, sometimes my focus will wander, and I'll find myself completely replicating the body language, posture, and energy level of one person. As soon as I notice I will usually return to my standard settings, standing straight and still with my arms crossed over my stomach, my energy low and my expression neutral. The victim of my mimicry will often look at me strangely and change his or her position to a guarded one, hands close together, eyes slightly wider, shoulders slightly slanted away from me, and both feet flat on the ground. I always feel bad when this happens, but of course I can't apologise as they would only feel more uncomfortable.

Some of my friends, however, find it hilarious. They think it's like a game, and they don't mind when things like this happen. These are the people I actually like spending time with. I don't consider talking to them a chore, unlike with any other people. That's because people like this understand how much I struggle with social interaction and take steps to make me feel more comfortable. They won't make eye contact unless I initiate it; they make their emotion clear and are explicit in their questions and requests. They won't ask, 'Imogen, do you want to wait at the bus stop with me?' They will instead say, 'Imogen, I want you to stay with me at the bus stop'. They let me know when there is a preferred answer by speaking like this, which makes me confident when agreeing or refusing. People like this mean that I have people outside my family that I can confide in and ask for advice from comfortably. They make my social life so much easier; it's hard to realise until you seriously consider who you want to be friends with and who you feel a duty to talk to.

Finally, I want to say that I like the fact that I'm autistic. But it is quite tiring to always be speaking a 'foreign – neuro-normal language', and I wish that occasionally the world spoke to me in my native tongue.

## Remember, it's a spectrum

Remember the quote at the beginning of this chapter:

> *If you have met one person with autism . . . you've met one person with autism.*
>
> Dr. Stephen Shore

This is so important to keep in mind. Just because they share a diagnosis, two children with ASD will likely present differently and have a different profile of strengths and needs.

The very nature of the spectrum means that children with ASD will have different abilities and difficulties. Remember also that children's skills will also be affected by any accompanying learning difficulty.

# Introduction to autism spectrum disorder (ASD)

Parents always ask, 'Where on the spectrum is he or she?' They want to know mild, moderate, severe, and so on. This can be a difficult question to answer; it's useful to think of a child's abilities and functional skills. ASD will impact them at different times across their lives. Also it doesn't necessarily follow that those who can talk have 'mild' ASD as the impact of the ASD can still be significant depending on the child.

No one knows what the future will bring; in the early years it is worth focussing on the present, therefore providing early intervention and giving the best start.

**RECAP** Now that you have read a lot of background information about ASD, you will understand that children with ASD have a complex communication profile and can present with varying needs. The very nature of the spectrum means that children will appear differently from each other. Their difficulties will present differently at different times in their lives.

**TIP** Keep an open mind, and remember that every child with ASD is different. All too often I've heard the following or similar statements many times. I've specifically included them here (see Figure 1.2) to illustrate that they aren't particularly helpful judgements to make about a child.

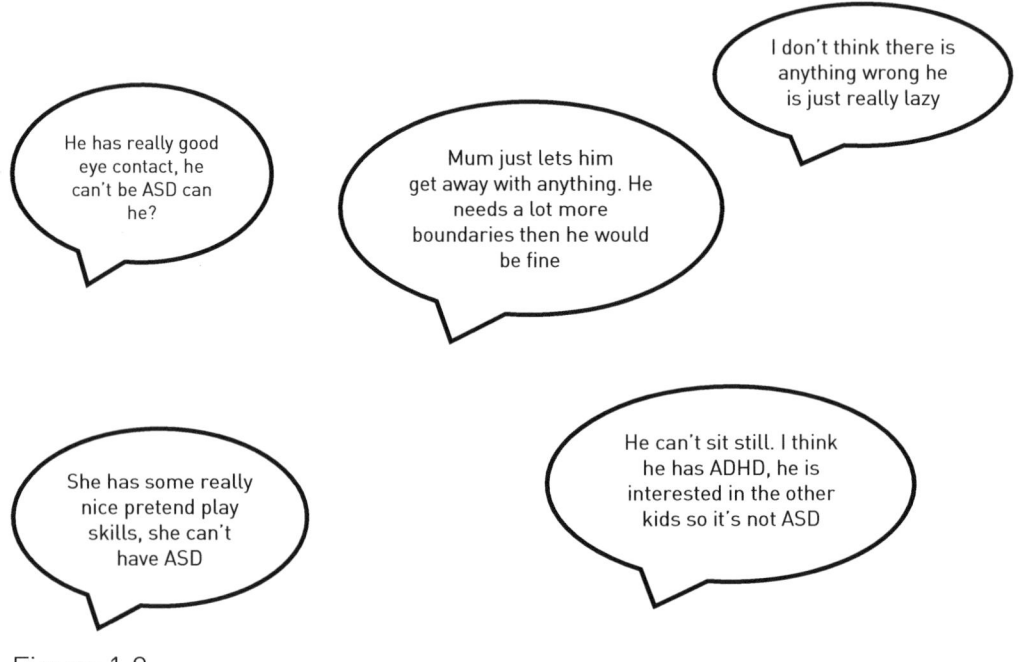

Figure 1.2

# Introduction to autism spectrum disorder (ASD)

Being a parent is hard work! I can only imagine that being a parent to a child with ASD comes with even more stress and challenges. We can support parents by being non-judgmental and sticking to objective observations about children rather than making comments and statements that at the time seem throwaway but can have a big impact.

Let's look at two examples to see how ASD can appear differently in young children. Both of these children have a diagnosis of ASD and have evident difficulties with their social communication and interaction and restricted and repetitive behaviours. However, the way these difficulties manifest is different for each child.

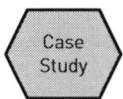

**Name:** Adam

**Age:** three years and six months

**About Adam**

- Adam received a diagnosis of ASD when he was two and a half.

- Staff working with him report that since getting the diagnosis he has made lots of progress. Having the diagnosis has been helpful because it means that they understand him more and have been able to access relevant training and support.

- Adam communicates using short phrases, for example, 'red square'. Most of his phrases are to label rather than to ask for things. Adam doesn't ask for things most of the time as he can get them himself or will take an adult's hand to the item.

- He knows the names of many items and frequently copies words.

- Adam understands the routine of the nursery but is unable to always respond to spoken instructions.

- Adam can be distracted and tends to only want to do his activity – he will spend hours playing with water and sand. His play with water and sand is repetitive, and he will do the same activity again and again, pouring between cups and a jug.

- Adam is interested in adults but does not show interest in his peers; often he will lean on other children or push them and laugh.

- Adam has some sensory difficulties, and he becomes distressed with certain noises including the cries of other children, a hand dryer, and adults singing. He will cover his ears and scream when these happen.

21

# Introduction to autism spectrum disorder (ASD)

**Strengths**

- Adam learns new words quickly.

- He is definitely interested in interacting with other people; he approaches others and watches them closely – but he doesn't seem to know what is appropriate.

- He focusses his attention on self-selected activities.

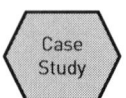

**Name:** Lucille

**Age:** four years and ten months

**About Lucille**

- Lucille is a bright and articulate young girl.

- Her nursery did not have any concerns about her skills until her parents shared their issues regarding her behaviour at home.

- Lucille recently received a diagnosis of ASD. At the time of diagnosis the diagnostic team described Lucille as 'high functioning' and similar to what would have been called 'Asperger's' in the past. The team also emphasised that girls with ASD present differently from boys. They drew attention to the fact that girls with ASD may 'mask' and 'internalise' some of their difficulties, which can cause anxiety.

- Lucille is verbal and talks in long sentences. She loves animals and will talk at length about these; she finds it difficult to have conversations with other people that aren't about animals.

- Lucille sometimes uses language that she has learnt from a book or television programme. She also has some slightly unusual phrases, for example, 'I do believe . . .' which gives her language a slightly formal quality.

- Lucille can become distressed if she thinks that a rule has been broken; she often will try to reinforce what she believes are rules which other children can find difficult. For example, within the nursery environment children are allowed only two minutes on a bike, which is shown by a timer. If a child stays on slightly longer, Lucille becomes distressed and tries to pull him or her off.

- Lucille tends to seek out adults.

- Lucille watches the other children closely.

# Introduction to autism spectrum disorder (ASD)

- Lucille can cope with the day-to-day routine at home and nursery but can find it difficult to cope with changes to the routine. There is a school trip coming up, and staff are worried how Lucille will cope with this.

**Strengths**

- Lucille has a strong sense of right and wrong.
- She has strong verbal communication.
- She would like a friend.

Although Adam and Lucille present with different features as part of their diagnoses, it is clear that they both have difficulties in the areas of social communication and interaction and restricted and repetitive behaviours.

*Activity* Think about Adam and Lucille's individual difficulties, and discuss as a group. Consider which characteristics may be related to social communication and interaction and which may be related to restricted and repetitive behaviours.

## What's it like to have ASD – the child's perspective

One of the reasons for writing this manual is a result of the wonderful children and families I have had the pleasure of working with. Alice, who has a diagnosis of ASD (age eight at the time of writing), has shared her insights as follows. When I asked her if she would be interested in sharing her experience, she suggested a question-and-answer format.

### What are you interested in?
*'I've had many obsessions before in life. First it was animals, then it was flags/capital cities, then cars, and now it is llamas'.*

### What do you find difficult?
*'I hate it when I get too hot or too cold. When this happens, I feel like shouting BAH very loudly'.*

### What are you good at?
*'I'm good at loads of things but mainly acting, remembering things, playing tunes I hear on my violin, singing, and running'.*

### What is autism?
*'Autism is something which makes someone different to normal people'.*

# Introduction to autism spectrum disorder (ASD)

**When did you find out about autism?**
*'How I found out was when my dad ran the marathon for the National Autistic Society'.*

**Is there anything that people do that helps you?**
*'Yes there is my mum and dad which help me. My teacher understands I am a bit different too'.*

**Is there anything that makes things tricky for you?**
*'I don't like it when I don't know what is going to happen and what I am supposed to do. I understand what people say literally – why am I asked to jump into bed or lay the table?'*

**Is there anything else you want to tell people reading this book?**
*'No'.*

Alice's and Imogen's insights give you an understanding of what it is like to have ASD. We will turn now to consider relevant theories relating to ASD.

Having an overview of the relevant theories is helpful in further developing your knowledge of ASD.

## Relevant theories

Understanding some of the key theories and perspectives related to ASD can help increase your understanding and further enable you to get into the shoes of a child with ASD. The following theories are useful to be aware of.

## Theory of mind

In its simplest sense theory of mind relates to understanding what other people are thinking and feeling. In 1985 Simon Baron Cohen, Uta Frith, and Alan Leslie suggested that children with ASD have difficulties with theory of mind.

Very young children don't typically understand that people see the world differently from themselves. In typical children the early stages of theory of mind start developing around age three and continue to develop until children are five. Theory of mind can develop at a different rate in typical children, but children with ASD are known to have difficulties with theory of mind that last much longer. Research shows that this is independent of IQ and intelligence.

In typical children theory of mind is one of the fundamentals of social understanding. Difficulties with theory of mind can have a huge impact on a child. Imagine not being able to make sense of another person's behaviour and communication? The world would seem confusing. Difficulties with theory of mind mean that children with ASD can find it difficult to understand that people may have a different view or perspective from them. This can also mean that children find it difficult to understand the feelings and thoughts of others.

## Central Coherence

Uta Frith described the Weak Central Coherence Theory of Autism in 1989. In its simplest sense Central Coherence is a term that means being able to see 'the bigger picture', as in the ability to draw meaning from lots of details. For example, a person with strong Central Coherence would be able to look at a room with balloons, a cake, and candles and describe 'a birthday party', but someone with weak Central Coherence would see the parts and not be able to draw meaning from it. This theory helps explain some of the strengths and difficulties experienced by people with ASD. An extreme focus on particular details can be difficult when you need to see the overall picture; however, it can lead to skills in certain areas, for example, mathematics or music.

## Executive dysfunction

Executive function relates to a range of cognitive processes that help us to regulate, control, and manage our thoughts and actions. These skills include memory, planning, attention, problem-solving, verbal reasoning, inhibition, cognitive flexibility, initiation of actions, and monitoring and regulating of actions. We need these skills for organising ourselves, being flexible, planning our actions, controlling our impulses, and being flexible. These skills are extremely important in many elements of everyday life.

One of the theories that seeks to explain the restricted and repetitive behaviours of people with a diagnosis of ASD is that of 'executive dysfunction'. Pennington and Ozonoff (1996) hypothesised that people with ASD have difficulties with executive function.

## The theory of empathising – systemising

The empathising–systemising (E-S) theory was developed by Simon Baron-Cohen (2002). This theory suggests that people can be classified on their scores on the Empathy Quotient and the Systemising Quotient.

## Introduction to autism spectrum disorder (ASD)

In its simplest terms the theory suggests that women tend to better at empathising (trying to understand the thoughts and feelings of others and respond appropriately to these) with men typically being better at systemising (seeking to make systems in a logical and systematic way). This theory is used to explain ASD insofar as people with ASD are also better at systemising with weaker skills in empathising. These concepts have also been used as part of the 'extreme male brain' (EMB) theory of ASD (Baron-Cohen, 2002).

## Understand the why

Having read this far in Chapter One by now, you will have a fairly good understanding of ASD.

You will know these main ideas:

- Children with ASD all present differently but will have difficulties across social communication and interaction and restricted and repetitive behaviours.
- Children with ASD may or may not have additional sensory difficulties.
- ASD may present differently in girls than boys.
- Children with ASD have many strengths.
- Each child with ASD is unique.

## Why is it important to know all this?

As we said at the beginning of this chapter; the more you can understand and 'get into the child's shoes', the more you can understand *why* a child is communicating or behaving in a certain way. This knowledge is crucial in enabling you to effectively plan and support children with ASD.

## Understanding ASD quiz

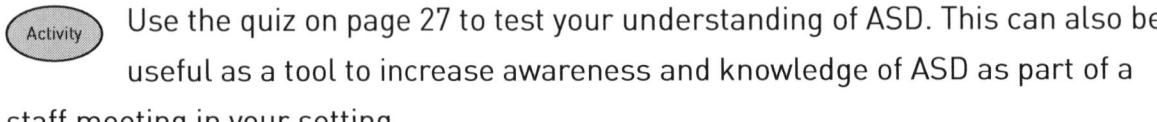

Use the quiz on page 27 to test your understanding of ASD. This can also be useful as a tool to increase awareness and knowledge of ASD as part of a staff meeting in your setting.

For answers to the quiz see Appendix One (page 195).

# Introduction to autism spectrum disorder (ASD)

**1** **ASD is a neurological and developmental disorder that children are born with**
TRUE/FALSE

**2** **People with ASD experience the world differently**
TRUE/FALSE

**3** **Children can grow out of ASD**
TRUE/FALSE

**4** **Once children can talk their ASD almost disappears**
TRUE/FALSE

**5** **There are more boys with ASD than girls**
TRUE/FALSE

**6** **How many people in the UK have ASD?**
One in 1000
One in 100
One in 10 000

**7** **Parents of children with ASD are to blame for their child's difficulties**
TRUE/FALSE

**8** **What two areas does a person need to have difficulties in to get a diagnosis of ASD?**

**9** **Vaccines cause ASD**
TRUE/FALSE

**10** **All people with ASD have sensory processing difficulties**
TRUE/FALSE

# Introduction to autism spectrum disorder (ASD)

## Getting a diagnosis

The process of getting a diagnosis of ASD can be quite long, both in terms of a waiting list but also in terms of parental readiness. Parents always know their child best, and whilst they may have a sense that there may be some aspects that are developing differently in their child, they may not be ready to consider a diagnosis. Even though parents may seem ready for the diagnosis, it can still be an extremely emotive and stressful process.

**TIP** Think of how you would feel if it was your child. When you are talking to parents or identifying difficulties, remember to describe a child's strengths as well as needs. If you are concerned about a child in your setting, remember the following:

- Talk to parents and ask them what happens at home. Often children can present differently in different situations, and this information can be helpful to know.

- Start with the positives: 'What's going well?'

- Record observations and planning; this documentation can be helpful when applying for support later on if it is required.

- Remember getting an ASD diagnosis is a process – leave the diagnosis to the child development team. I've heard 'He's definitely got autism' many times. Whilst a child may have many features and may get a diagnosis, it's not helpful to label without a diagnosis.

- See the child, not the label.

- If a parent asks you questions that you don't know the answer to, don't feel tempted to say something misleading like, 'Don't worry . . . he will be fine'.

- Signpost parents to local speech and language therapy services. Encourage parents to go to their general practitioner and discuss their concerns.

- Unfortunately there is a lot of misleading information on the internet about ASD which can lead to parents going away feeling confused and upset. Recommending the previously mentioned websites is a good place to start.

- If your area has a local child development service, find out what the process is in terms of making a referral and who can do this. If you are able to provide this information to parents in a timely way, this can be supportive.

# Introduction to autism spectrum disorder (ASD)

A paediatrician, speech and language therapist, or clinical psychologist is usually involved in the assessment. The assessment will likely involve direct observation and assessment with the child, a structured parental history, and possibly an observation in a different context such as a nursery. For more information about ASD assessments and the process involved, see The National Autistic Society, which provides a useful outline.

## Getting a diagnosis – a parent's perspective

Listening to the experiences of parents of children with ASD is a useful and important way of understanding more about the process and how we as health-care professionals and educators can best support. A wonderful parent who I have worked with, Becky, mother to four children all with ASD traits kindly agreed to share her experiences.

### *Challenges*

One of the biggest challenges as a parent both pre- and post-diagnosis was simply the lack of knowledge in the education system. Having four children, all with elements of the autistic spectrum, and one with an actual diagnosis of ASD, I have spent a lot of time trying to explain (and at times persuade) educationalists that my children have additional needs. Because my children are all 'high functioning', the subtleties of their autism has often made it hard for teachers to understand or even believe the symptoms. At preschool age my children's sensory processing difficulties would be dismissed as 'tantrums', and their poor conversation skills passed off as 'a shy child'. As a mum I always knew they were different, but often felt I was having to convince those around me.

Even in the health system, I have found that the criteria for diagnosis only goes so far. A low-functioning child is obviously easier to recognise, but in my case, I had 'little professors' whose language skills were overdeveloped so they never ticked a box for 'speaking late'. Equally, despite their frequent meltdowns at home, they would often conform in a nursery or school environment, so their challenging behaviours weren't observed. I think two of my children were probably 'missed' and should have received diagnoses when they were three. I would have appreciated more knowledge of how high-functioning children operated, and their hidden difficulties, both in the health and education system.

One other frustration that I continually experienced was that every interview I had with a health professional needed me to have my child with me. With highly intelligent and

## Introduction to autism spectrum disorder (ASD)

sensitive children, it felt so wrong speaking about their challenging behaviours while they were present. I eventually learnt to always have another adult with me so they could take my child out. I think the initial contact with a parent, who will be inevitably stressed and often emotional, would ideally be without the child. It would give the parent a chance to speak freely and openly without worrying about what the child is hearing.

### *Diagnosis and support*

I have experienced first-hand the postcode lottery around diagnosis and support. In West London, I took three of my children through multidisciplinary assessments. Following one of my son's diagnosis for ASD, the support was overwhelming. I thought this must be normal. I had no idea how lucky I was! He had instant speech language therapist (SLT), OT, and a psychologist. At one point he even had music therapy on the NHS. My biggest stress was trying to implement the various strategies I was given for him while also managing my other sensory and socially challenged children. Then I moved to Birmingham. My support went to zero. In four years I have received nothing on the NHS for any of my children. It has been unbelievably hard, and I feel the system has failed my children. My son became violent and very oppositional after a year in Birmingham, and it took two full years to get an appointment with CAMHS. Once he was finally assessed, no therapy was given. Despite writing to MPs and local paediatricians, the money is not here for autistic children. Friends of mine with newly diagnosed autistic children have received absolutely no therapeutic input. I have been stunned at the difference!

### *Tips for parents with nursery-age children*

- In my experience this is the toughest age, and it will get easier as your child gets older! Whether it's toilet training, social skills, or meltdowns, generally with age, the stress will ease, and your child will learn. I found two to three years such a hard age for autism.

- The transition to nursery is helpful if you can put together a visual book and timetable. It helped my children to see pictures of their key workers and the rooms they would play in. We looked at these a lot before they started. As much as possible make things feel familiar. Change is so stressful for children with autism at this age.

- Gentle exposure is a good strategy for helping your little one handle the change. My youngest child was unbearably unhappy at the start of nursery, so I started with a half-hour separation and then increased it gradually. I have used gentle exposure for so many of my children's fears: clothing, toilet training, sleep, and so on. I've learnt to take things slowly and not expect too much too soon. It demands patience, but the results are worth it – even if your child is in nappies until they are four or five! It's not the end of the world!

- The best thing I learnt through our child psychologist in London was that when my preschooler had a meltdown or showed challenging behaviour, he or she wasn't trying to communicate something. I couldn't always work out what they needed, but it helped to lower my stress level and stopped me getting angry when I realised they were showing me through their screams that they felt sad or frustrated or scared.

Finally, it has been said that a parent with an autistic child has a stress level comparable to a combat soldier. I think everyone involved in this field needs to remember that the mothers and fathers they are working with are vulnerable. They will be tired, stressed, often anxious or depressed, and desperate for validation and help. They need to hear that no parent is equipped to cope with these challenges. They need to know that they are doing the best they can. And they need their health and education professionals to be voices of strength and hope.

## *After diagnosis*

Post-diagnostic support will vary dependent upon your geographical location, as highlighted by Becky's experiences. Many areas will run a parent workshop or group that can be informative.

The following programmes provide practical activities and support. They may run in your area and can be useful to signpost parents to:

- EarlyBird (under age five years) and EarlyBird Plus (aged four–nine) are programmes for parents and carers of children with ASD. For more information see www.autism.org/earlybird

- More than Words®–The Hanen Program® for Parents of Children with Autism Spectrum Disorder or Social Communication Difficulties is a programme run by

# Introduction to autism spectrum disorder (ASD)

Hanen-certified SLTs all over the world. In addition to the taught programme, the guide book is an extremely useful resource (detailed in references).

These programmes all require a licensed practitioner to run the course, so depending on the provision in your area, there may be something different on offer. Regardless of what is available, meeting and connecting with other parents can be helpful and supportive.

In addition to specific post-diagnostic groups, most areas have parent support groups either via the National Autistic Society or other local parent groups.

Get in touch with your local services to find out what is on offer to ensure that parents are able to access what they are entitled to.

## Let's get started!

Now that you have a good understanding of ASD, let's get started in using this manual. This manual provides two tools to help you learn more about children in your setting.

These tools are designed to help you make useful observations and gather relevant information to support goal setting and progress.

Depending on where you live, a child with ASD's access to services may vary hugely. In reality this means that some children start an education environment with a diagnosis and support in place, whereas other children may start without a diagnosis or referral to any relevant professionals. Gathering information and documenting it is of key importance to tracking progress, which is important when it comes to getting further specific support, for example, an Education Health Care Plan. The Skills Profile (I-1) and Information-Gathering Tool (I-2) are useful to start observing the children you work with and to help you gather relevant information about the children you work with. See pages 40–41 for blank copies of the Skills Profile and Information-Gathering Tool.

## *I-1: the Skills Profile*

The profile helps you make observations of where a child is in terms of his or her skills. Talking about a child's strengths and needs in terms of a profile can be helpful in explaining development. Often children that I have worked with have shown strengths in certain areas and needs in others that do not follow a linear and typical pattern. Using the profile helps you think of using a child's strengths to build on his or her needs. You can complete the Skills Profile at different time points through the year as a progress tool or use it as an assessment tool. The profile offers a 'snapshot' of skills at a particular time. See page 40 for a blank copy of the Skills Profile.

*Note that the tool does not follow a developmental progression – it does not go through each stage in a developmental sequence. This reflects the atypical pattern of communication that children with ASD have.

## I-2: the Information-Gathering Tool

The tool helps you to make observations that can support discussion with parents in addition to a starting place for target setting. See page 41 for a blank copy of the Information-Gathering Tool.

Let's revisit our earlier case studies, Adam and Lucille, to look at their completed Skills Profiles and Information-Gathering Tools; these provide examples of how the tools may be used to break down strengths and needs. Turn now to the following pages for examples.

## Skills Profile:

| Name: | Adam |
|---|---|
| Date: | 4.5.2018 |
| Completed by: | Jennifer Warwick |

| Stage of attention (Adapted from Reynell et al.) | Understanding | Communication checklist | Play | Social interaction |
|---|---|---|---|---|
| **Level one** – Very distractible with fleeting attention only | - Does not understand words<br>- Does not understand gestures<br>- Shows understanding of some familiar routines, e.g., shoes, going out ✓<br>- Responds to a few key words, e.g., 'no', 'snack' ✓<br>- Responds to gestures, e.g., knows waving means bye-bye | **Non-verbal**<br>- Reaches<br>- Makes sounds (no meaning)<br>- Makes sounds (with meaning, e.g., brum for car)<br>- Points to ask<br>- Points to share interest<br>- Communicative eye contact<br>- Gives items<br>- Becomes frustrated if unable to communicate ✓<br>- Uses your hand ✓<br>- Pulls to items ✓<br>Turns away to say no<br>Pushes away to say no<br>**Gestures**<br>- Wave<br>- Hands up<br>- Finished<br>- Push away<br>- Nods head<br>- Shakes head<br>- Other<br>**Verbal**<br>- Single words ✓<br>- Phrases<br>- Verbs<br>- Sentences<br>**Functions**<br>- Requests – objects<br>- Labels ✓ Protests<br>- Requests – social<br>- Comments<br>- Greets<br>- Questions<br>- Shares information | **Exploratory**<br>Explores objects with senses, e.g., mouthing, listening, watching ✓ | - Does not appear to notice others<br>- Does not make any attempts to interact<br>- Child mostly in his or her own world<br>- Watches others but does not join in ✓<br>- Plays alongside other children ✓<br>- Engages in shared attention ✓ |
| **Level two** – Attends to own choice of activity for a longer period of time but cuts self off from everything else ✓ | | | **Cause and effect**<br>Enjoys the impact of their actions and understands they make things happen, e.g., pop-up toy, banging a drum ✓ | - Shows shared enjoyment<br>- Joins in a familiar game or song (e.g., 'Row, Row, Row Your Boat' with an adult<br>- Joins in a familiar game or song (e.g., 'Row, Row, Row Your Boat' with another child<br>- Can join in a group game, e.g., parachute, 'What's the Time, Mr Wolf'<br>- Enjoys being with others ✓<br>- Starts a game, e.g., chase or tickle<br>- Asks for a turn, 'My turn' |
| **Level three** – Still single-channelled attention but begins to attend to adults | - Can follow instructions in context, e.g., 'Come here', 'Sit down'<br>- Shows understanding of everyday familiar vocabulary, e.g., toys, body parts, etc. | | **Functional play**<br>Understands the conventional function of objects, e.g., filling a container, building a tower | - Controls play and becomes upset if it is not the way he or she wants<br>- Can wait for a turn as part of a structured game |
| **Level four** – Still single-channelled but able to shift attention between tasks with prompts | - Understands action words, e.g., jump, run, sleep, eat<br>- Understands short instructions:<br>(1) with two parts, 'Give me the spoon and the teddy' (where there are alternatives)<br>(2) with three key parts, 'Give me ball, apple, and cup' (where there are alternatives)<br>- Understands questions (circle), what, who, where, when, why | | **Early pretend play**<br>*Self-pretend* – brushes hair, holds toy phone to ear<br>*Other pretend* – feeds teddy, brushes doll | - Attempts to initiate social interaction with others (adult/child) may not be appropriate (list how the child does this, e.g., touches, gives, etc.)<br>- Attempts to initiate social interaction with others (adult/child) appropriately<br>- In structured, familiar activities |
| **Level five** – Integrated attention for short periods of time | | | **Imaginative play**<br>Uses items and self imaginatively | - In unstructured times |
| **Level six** – Integrated attention well established | | | **Co-operative play**<br>✓Engages in play activities with peers | - Two-way interaction (will respond to and initiate with others as part of a structured sequence):<br>- In a structured activity<br>- During unstructured times |

# Information Gathering:

| Name: | Adam |
|---|---|
| Date: | 4.5.2018 |
| Completed by: | Jennifer Warwick |

| Date | Information gathering | Notes | Other observations: It can be useful to make observations during particular activities as detailed. Step back and write down what the child does at the following times. |
|---|---|---|---|
| | **Sensory:**<br>– Any sensory sensitivities (noise, touch, environment)<br>– Sensory preferences (what do they like): movement, sound, visual | Adam can find certain noises distressing, e.g., crying, hand dryer, and singing | **Snack time:**<br>– Will sit for snack<br>– Enjoys snack time and watches others |
| | **Areas of strength:**<br>Find out from parents as well as your observations | – Focus on activities that he likes<br>– Likes to figure out how things work<br>– Persistent<br>– Good sense of humour<br>– Learns new words | **Free play:**<br>– Tends to wander around the room<br>– Will focus on water and sand for a long time |
| | **Areas of need:**<br>Find out from parents as well as your observations | – Asking for things<br>– Coping with changes | **Small groups:**<br>– Unable to join in |
| | **Best time of day:**<br>Is there a particular time of day that is best? Reflect on why this could be. How does child behave, communicate, or interact at this time that is different from other times? | After nap time Adam always seems more receptive | **Large groups (including circle time):**<br>– Unable to join in |
| | **Parental/carer priority:**<br>What would parents/carers like to work on?<br>What would make a difference to parent/carer and child? | – Toilet training and behaviour<br>– Being less frustrated and asking for things more | **Transitions:**<br>Attention is self-directed, tends to only want to do his own thing, will have a meltdown if he needs to move onto other activities that he is not interested in |
| | **Staff priority:**<br>What would staff like to work on?<br>What would make a difference to staff and child? | – Reduce Adam's frustration<br>– Following instructions<br>– Focussing on tasks | **Other:** |

# Skills Profile:

| Name: | Lucille |
|---|---|
| Date: | 4.5.2018 |
| Completed by: | Jennifer Warwick |

| Stage of attention (Adapted from Reynell et al.) | Understanding | Communication checklist | Play | Social interaction |
|---|---|---|---|---|
| **Level one** – Very distractible with fleeting attention only | – Does not understand words<br>– Does not understand gestures<br>– Shows understanding of some familiar routines, e.g., shoes on means going out<br>– Responds to a few key words, e.g., 'no', 'snack'<br>– Responds to gestures, e.g., knows waving means bye-bye ✓<br>– Can follow instructions in context, e.g., 'Come here', 'Sit down' ✓<br>– Shows understanding of everyday familiar vocabulary, e.g., toys, body parts etc. ✓<br>– Understands action words, e.g., jump, run, sleep, eat ✓<br>– Understands short instructions:<br>(1) with two parts, 'Give me the spoon and the teddy' (where there are alternatives) ✓<br>(2) with three key parts, 'Give me ball, apple, and cup' (where there are alternatives)<br>– Understands questions: what ✓, who ✓, where ✓, when, why | **Nonverbal**<br>– Reaches<br>– Makes sounds (no meaning)<br>– Makes sounds (with meaning, e.g., brum for car)<br>– Points to ask<br>– Points to share interest<br>– Communicative eye contact<br>– Gives items<br>– Becomes frustrated if unable to communicate<br>– Uses your hand<br>– Pulls to items<br>– Turns away to say no<br>– Pushes away to say no<br>**Gestures**<br>– Wave ✓<br>– Hands up<br>– Finished<br>– Push away<br>– Nods head ✓<br>– Shakes head ✓<br>– Other<br>**Verbal**<br>– Single words ✓<br>– Phrases ✓<br>– Verbs ✓<br>– Sentences ✓<br>**Functions**<br>– Requests – objects<br>– Labels ✓<br>– Protests<br>– Requests –social<br>– Comments ✓<br>– Greets<br>– Questions<br>– Shares information | **Exploratory**<br>Explores objects with senses, e.g., mouthing, listening, watching | – Does not appear to notice others<br>– Does not make any attempts to interact<br>– Child mostly in his or her own world<br>– Watches others but does not join in ✓<br>– Plays alongside other children ✓<br>– Engages in shared attention ✓<br>– Shows shared enjoyment ✓<br>– Joins in a familiar game or song (e.g., 'Row, Row, Row Your Boat' with an adult ✓ |
| **Level two** – Attends to own choice of activity for a longer period of time but cuts self off from everything else | | | **Cause and effect**<br>Enjoys the impact of their actions and understands they make things happen, e.g., pop-up toy, banging a drum | – Joins in a familiar game or song (e.g., 'Row, Row, Row Your Boat' with another child<br>– Can join in a group game, e.g., parachute, 'What's the Time, Mr Wolf' ✓ |
| **Level three** – Still single-channelled attention but begins to attend to adults ✓ | | | **Functional play**<br>Understands the conventional function of objects, e.g., filling a container, building a tower | – Enjoys being with others<br>– Starts a game, e.g., chase or tickle<br>– Asks for a turn, 'My turn'<br>– Controls play and becomes upset if it is not the way they want. ✓ |
| **Level four** – Still single-channelled but able to shift attention between tasks with prompts | | | **Early pretend play**<br>*Self-pretend* – brushes hair, holds toy phone to ear<br>*Other pretend* – feeds teddy, brushes doll | – Can wait for a turn as part of a structured game<br>– Attempts to initiate social interaction with others (adult/child) may not be appropriate (list how the child does this, e.g., touches, gives, etc.)<br>– Attempts to initiate social interaction with others (adult/child) appropriately<br>– In structured, familiar activities |
| **Level five** – Integrated attention for short periods of time | | | **Imaginative play**<br>Uses items and self imaginatively | |
| **Level six** – Integrated attention well established | | | **Co-operative play**<br>Engages in play activities with peers | – In unstructured times<br>– Two-way interaction (will respond to and initiate with others as part of a structured sequence):<br>– In a structured activity<br>– During unstructured times - |

## Information Gathering:

| Name: | Lucille |
|---|---|
| Date: | 4.5.2018 |
| Completed by: | Jennifer Warwick |

| Date | Information gathering | Notes | Other observations: It can be useful to make observations during particular activities as detailed. Step back and write down what the child does at the following times. |
|---|---|---|---|
| | **Sensory:**<br>- Any sensory sensitivities (noise, touch, environment)<br>- Sensory preferences (what do they like): movement, sound, visual | Lucille does not like messy play | **Snack time:**<br>- Walks around rather than sitting with a group<br>- Enjoys helping |
| | **Areas of strength:**<br>Find out from parents as well as your observations | - Verbal communication<br>- Vocabulary<br>- Imitation skills<br>- Interested in others<br>- Wants to engage and interact | **Free play:**<br>Can seem 'lost' during free-play activities, watches other children but does not approach them or engage and tends to gravitate to adults |
| | **Areas of need:**<br>Find out from parents as well as your observations | Difficulty in requesting – Lucille does not ask for help, e.g., will say, 'It's stuck' instead of 'Help me'; she does not always direct her communication to others; unable to start interactions or ask others to play | **Small groups:**<br>Tends to enjoy small-group sessions |
| | **Best time of day:**<br>Is there a particular time of day that is best, reflect on why this could be, how does child behave, communicate, or interact at this time that is different from other times? | Mornings are much better | **Large groups (including circle time):**<br>Dependent on her level of interest, if not interested will just walk away |
| | **Parental/carer priority:**<br>What would parents/carers like to work on?<br>What would make a difference to parent/carer and child? | Parents are keen for Lucille to be able to take turns and share as she snatches items from her younger sibling at home; they would like her to have a friend | **Transitions:**<br>Very distressed at transition times if there is a transition out of the nursery environment |
| | **Staff priority:**<br>What would staff like to work on?<br>What would make a difference to staff and child? | Transitions<br>Peer relationships | **Other:** |

# Introduction to autism spectrum disorder (ASD)

## Chapter One summary

- Although children with ASD will all present differently, they will all share common difficulties with social interaction and communication and restricted and repetitive behaviours. These may manifest in different ways depending on the child.

- Girls with ASD may present differently from boys.

- Many children with ASD, but not all, have sensory difficulties.

- Children with ASD have poor theory of mind – this means that they don't develop an understanding of how other people are thinking and feeling in the same way as other children.

- Difficulties with central coherence means that children with ASD can focus on the smaller details and struggle to see and understand the whole picture.

- Difficulties with executive functioning mean that children with ASD may show difficulties with planning, organisation, and impulse control.

- Chapter One has introduced you to the Skills Profile and Information-Gathering Tool which you will use to gather observations about children that you work with and as a planning tool. Start thinking about children in your setting and plotting them on the profile.

## References

American Psychiatric Association (2013). *Diagnostic and Statistical Manual of Mental Disorders: Diagnostic and Statistical Manual of Mental Disorders*, Fifth Edition. Arlington, VA: American Psychiatric Association.

Baron-Cohen, S. (2002). The extreme male brain theory of autism. *TRENDS in Cognitive Science*, 6(6), 248–256.

Baron-Cohen, S., Leslie, A. M. and Frith, U. (1985). Does the autistic child have a "theory of mind"? *Cognition*, 21, 37–46.

Biel, L. and Peske, N. (2009). *Raising a Sensory Smart Child: The Definitive Handbook for Helping Your Child with Sensory Processing Issues*. USA: Penguin Books.

Frith, U. (1989). *Autism: Explaining the Enigma*. Oxford: Blackwell.

Pennington, B. F. and Ozonoff, S. (1996). Executive functions and developmental psychopathology. *Journal of Child Psychology and Psychiatry and Allied Disciplines*, 37(1), 51–87.

Stock Kranowitz, C. (2005). *The Out of Sync Child: Recognizing and Coping with Sensory Processing Disorder*. USA: Penguin Books.

Sussman, F. (2012). *More Than Words®: A Parent's Guide to Building Interaction and Language Skills for Children with Autism Spectrum Disorder or Social Communication Difficulties*. Toronto, Ontario: The Hanen Centre.

# Skills Profile:

**Name:**

**Date:**

**Completed by:**

| Stage of attention (Adapted from Reynell et al) | Understanding | Communication checklist: (tick all that apply) | Play | Social interaction (tick all that apply) |
|---|---|---|---|---|
| **Level one** – Very distractible with fleeting attention only | – Does not understand words<br>– Does not understand gestures<br>– Shows understanding of some familiar routines, e.g., shoes on means going out | **Nonverbal**<br>– Reaches<br>– Makes sounds (no meaning)<br>– Makes sounds (with meaning, e.g., brum for car)<br>– Points to ask | **Exploratory**<br>Explores objects with senses, e.g., mouthing, listening, watching | – Does not appear to notice others<br>– Does not make any attempts to interact<br>– Child mostly in his or her own world<br>– Watches others but does not join in<br>– Plays alongside other children |
| **Level two** – Attends to own choice of activity for a longer period of time but cuts self off from everything else | – Responds to a few key words, e.g., 'no', 'snack'<br>– Responds to gestures e.g. knows waving means bye-bye | – Points to share interest<br>– Communicative eye contact<br>– Gives items<br>– Becomes frustrated if unable to communicate<br>– Uses your hand<br>– Pulls to items | **Cause and effect**<br>Enjoys the impact of their actions and understands they make things happen, e.g., pop-up toy, banging a drum | – Engages in shared attention<br>– Shows shared enjoyment<br>– Joins in a familiar game or song (e.g., 'Row, Row, Row Your Boat' with an adult<br>– Joins in a familiar game or song (e.g., 'Row, Row, Row Your Boat' with another child |
| **Level three** – Still single-channelled attention but begins to attend to adults | – Can follow instructions in context, e.g., 'Come here', 'Sit down'<br>– Shows understanding of everyday familiar vocabulary, e.g., toys, body parts, etc. | – Turns away to say no<br>– Pushes away to say no<br>**Gestures**<br>– Wave<br>– Hands up<br>– Finished<br>– Push away | **Functional play**<br>Understands the conventional function of objects, e.g., filling a container, building a tower | – Can join in a group game, e.g., parachute, 'What's the Time, Mr Wolf'<br>– Enjoys being with others<br>– Starts a game, e.g., chase or tickle<br>– Asks for a turn, 'My turn'<br>– Controls play and becomes upset if it is not the way they want |
| **Level four** – Still single-channelled but able to shift attention between tasks with prompts | – Understands action words, e.g., jump, run, sleep, eat<br>– Understands short instructions:<br>(1) with two parts, 'Give me the spoon and the teddy' (where there are alternatives)<br>(2) with three key parts, 'Give me ball, apple, and cup' (where there are alternatives) | – Nods head<br>– Shakes head<br>– Other<br>**Verbal**<br>– Single words<br>– Phrases<br>– Verbs<br>– Sentences | **Early pretend play**<br>*Self-pretend* – brushes hair, holds toy phone to ear<br>*Other pretend* – feeds teddy, brushes doll | – Can wait for a turn as part of a structured game<br>– Attempts to initiate social interaction with others (adult/child) may not be appropriate (list how the child does this, e.g., touches, gives, etc.) |
| **Level five** – Integrated attention for short periods of time | – Understands questions (circle), what, who, where, when, why | **Functions**<br>– Requests – objects<br>– Labels<br>– Protests<br>– Requests – social<br>– Comments<br>– Greets<br>– Questions<br>– Shares information | **Imaginative play**<br>Uses items and self imaginatively | – Attempts to initiate social interaction with others (adult/child) appropriately<br>– In structured familiar activities<br>– In unstructured times |
| **Level six** – Integrated attention well established | | | **Co-operative play**<br>Engages in play activities with peers | – Two-way interaction (will respond to and initiate with others as part of a structured sequence):<br>– In a structured activity<br>– During unstructured times |

Copyright material from Jennifer Warwick (2020) *Supporting SLCN in Children with ASD in the Early Years*, Routledge

# Information Gathering:

**Name:**

**Date:**

**Completed by:**

| Date | Information gathering | Notes |
|---|---|---|
| | **Sensory:**<br>- Any sensory sensitivities (noise, touch, environment)<br>- Sensory preferences (what do they like): movement, sound, visual | |
| | **Areas of strength:**<br>Find out from parents as well as your observations | |
| | **Areas of need:**<br>Find out from parents as well as your observations | |
| | **Best time of day:**<br>Is there a particular time of day that is best, reflect on why this could be, how does child behave, communicate, or interact at this time that is different from other times? | |
| | **Parental/carer priority:**<br>What would parents/carers like to work on?<br>What would make a difference to parent/carer and child? | |
| | **Staff priority:**<br>What would staff like to work on?<br>What would make a difference to staff and child? | |

**Other observations:**
It can be useful to make observations during particular activities as detailed. Step back and write down what the child does at the following times.

| Snack time: |
| Free play: |
| Small groups: |
| Large groups (including circle time): |
| Transitions: |
| Other: |

Copyright material from Jennifer Warwick (2020) *Supporting SLCN in Children with ASD in the Early Years*, Routledge

# Chapter Two
# THE EARLY YEARS ENVIRONMENT: CHALLENGES AND OPPORTUNITIES

**Chapter Two provides the following:**

- An overview of the challenges in the early years environment

- Strategies to overcome these challenges using the strengths of children with ASD

- Strategies on how we can increase understanding in the early years environment through use of visual supports, routines, and structured teaching

- Activity sheets:

    **(E1) – Using objects to support understanding**

    **(E2) – Using photos to help understanding**

    **(E3) – Using a first/then board**

    **(E4) – Understanding the concept 'finished' and using a countdown**

    **(E5) – Using a visual timetable**

    **(E6) – Understanding the concept of 'wait' and using a wait card**

    **(E7) – Using visuals to support independence in everyday activities**

    **(E8) – Language for routines**

    **(E9) – Structuring the education environment – let's make a plan**

# The early years environment

- **(E10) – Structuring the learning environment – top tips**
- **(E11) – Structuring a one-on-one area using a workstation**
- **(E12) – Structuring one-on-one activities**
- **(E13) – Managing changes in the routine**

## Early years education

Starting in education can be a daunting prospect for all parents and their children. These feelings may be amplified for a parent of a child with ASD and in fact any Special Educational Need or Disability (SEND) or SLCN. Whilst early years education is crucial for children with ASD, the environment itself can be stressful and overwhelming.

New people, sounds, smells, routines, and unclear expectations can all be huge challenges to overcome and understand for the child with ASD. From your reading of relevant theories in Chapter One, you can understand some of the challenges children and young people with ASD face in an education environment.

Ensuring that the start to an education environment is successful can have a huge impact on a child, the family, and also the staff working with the child.

The good news is there is lots that can be done to support a child with ASD entering nursery to ensure optimal success.

Preparation and understanding are key factors. Many of the most successful placements and transitions for children with ASD I have seen have hinged on this. In many cases these have been early years settings with no prior experience of children with ASD; however, a willingness and commitment to learn makes all the difference.

In this chapter we look at the challenges and the opportunities within the environment and work through how you can adapt your setting to best support a child with ASD.

**TIP** In my work as an SLT I have been lucky to work with wonderful educators and health-care professionals. Some of the key principles emphasised by

# The early years environment

these wonderful people have stuck with me and can be top tips for anyone working with a child with ASD. Keeping these in your mind as guiding principles can be a useful starting point.

> *Change yourself . . . not the child.*
> *Show me, don't tell me.*
> *Always strengths first.*
> *Bring structure to the unstructured.*
> *Be prepared.*

## Challenges within the environment

Early years environments can be overwhelming for children with ASD.

The free flow curriculum can mean that children with ASD can become more self-directed, focussing for long periods on activities of their own choosing. Whilst initially this can appear as if a child is happy playing, this can present later as a difficulty as it becomes increasingly difficult to get them to focus on other areas and activities, especially those that an adult wants them to focus on.

In Chapter One we talked about the sensory challenges that some children with ASD may experience. If you think about your environment, consider the challenges in terms of external stimulation, noises, and visual and tactile information. These factors may all be difficult for a child to process and cope with.

Whilst early years environments may follow a routine there can be changes to this, and at times the unpredictable nature of what is happening during the day, which typically developing children just take in their stride, can be difficult to manage.

Often I see children having 'meltdowns' with staff unsure why or what has happened to trigger this. In many cases, through discussion and observation we are able to work out that a factor in the environment has caused this to happen.

Whilst there are many challenges in the environment and the inevitable problem of not always enough staff to implement changes 'just for one child', there is a lot that can be done to overcome these challenges.

## So with all of these challenges, what can we do to help?

**TIP** Making changes to the environment can seem like a lot of work for 'just one child'. Try not to think about it like this as the changes you make will support all the children in your setting including those with other SEND or SLCN and children with English as an additional language (EAL). Recognise that making changes does take time and works best when everyone signs up to the challenge.

I have worked within settings that have implemented changes to the environment and then discarded them after they haven't worked after a week. Think how long it takes to change any behaviour in an adult or a child; make sure that you give enough time (at least a half term) to allow for change.

Using your knowledge of ASD and showing awareness as to why a child may be experiencing difficulties in the environment is helpful in itself. Sadly all too often I have worked with parents when they have felt people judging or even worse commenting on how their child responds in situations, for example, on the bus, whilst waiting in the shopping queue, or on a visit to a hospital. Acknowledging that different environments can be difficult for a child with ASD is important. Going back to Becky's insights as a parent highlights how, as health-care professionals and educators, we need to be non-judgmental, supportive, and most of all, listening.

## Overcoming challenges by using a child's strengths

Using the strengths of children with ASD is a great way to support them in the early years environment. It also has the bonus of focussing on what a child can do as opposed to what they can't.

We mentioned the strengths of children with ASD in Chapter One. Here we look in more detail at how we can use these strengths in a positive way.

### *Children with ASD are visual learners*

'*Show me don't just tell me*' is a mantra many SLTs and specialist teachers live by.

Spoken words are transient, and often children with ASD seem to not be able to take on spoken information. If you can show children what is happening visually as well as using gestures and spoken words, they are much more likely to understand. In the same way as when we are learning a foreign language, we benefit from the use of pictures, gestures, and seeing the object that is being spoken about, so too do children with ASD.

Many interventions for children with ASD use visuals as a key part. It makes sense to use a child's strengths as a starting point. We know that children with ASD have strengths in their visual learning, so we can use visual supports to enable their communication.

## What are visual supports?

Firstly, it is helpful to clarify the difference in using visuals to help a child understand and using visuals to support expressive communication. I have visited many settings where all visual supports have been referred to as 'PECS'. PECS stands for the picture exchange communication system and is an alternative and augmentative system developed in 1985 in the United States. This is a highly structured approach introduced to support a child's ability to make requests. PECS is typically introduced by the therapist and requires daily practise.

For more information regarding the Picture Exchange communication system see www.pecs.org.uk.

Using visual supports is different from PECS. Visual supports can be useful to help a child make a request or a choice or send you a message (expressive communication). We also use visual supports to help understanding (receptive communication), for example, a timetable, first-next board, or photographs. This chapter focusses on using visual supports for understanding; we will look in more detail at visual supports for expressive communication in Chapter Three.

Visual supports can be objects, pictures, photos, and miniature objects. The key part is that they are permanent, unlike a spoken word or gesture which once spoken or signed disappears. Using visual supports provides extra information alongside the spoken word to help a child understand. I have found there is the added extra that using the visual support tends to slow down an adult's talking which will also help a child's understanding.

We all use visual supports in our daily lives to help us complete tasks and understand information. Think of your to-do list or cooking something new from a recipe book, or imagine being in a foreign country where you may find it hard to understand and speak the language. You would likely be reliant on visual cues around you to help you understand; you might point to a map or sign or show a picture in your guidebook. These are all similar to using visuals to support communication.

It is important to be aware that some visual supports are easier to understand than others. Whether to use an object, picture, or symbol should depend on each individual child's learning style and understanding.

Objects are generally viewed as the easiest to understand. This relates to a child's developmental stage and is known as symbolic representation. The more concrete the visual support, the easier it is to understand; for example, showing a nappy each time a child is going to be changed is easier to comprehend than looking at a picture of a nappy. The hierarchy of symbolic representation from easiest to hardest to understand is shown as follows. It is useful to bear this in mind as all too often we start using symbols when actually a child may not be ready for these.

**Hierarchy of symbolic representation**

**EASIEST TO UNDERSTAND**
- REAL OBJECT
- MINATURE OBJECT
- PHOTOGRAPH
- LINE DRAWING
- SYMBOL
- WRITTEN WORD

**HARDEST TO UNDERSTAND**

> **TIP** Avoid images such as cartoons and those that you may find on clip art. These can be confusing for children.

Ensure that any visuals used at home are the same as those in the education setting. It could be confusing for a child to have different systems at home and nursery.

# The early years environment

One of the most portable and easily accessible ways to provide visuals (if a child is able to understand line drawings) is to use a wipe-clean whiteboard and draw the visual supports. This has the added bonus of being portable and easy for parents to also use so there is continuity between the education environment and home.

Turn now to the following activity sheets for practical ideas on supporting understanding in a visual way.

**(E1) – Using objects to support understanding**
**(E2) – Using photos to help understanding**
**(E3) – Using a first/then board**
**(E4) – Understanding the concept 'finished' and using a countdown**
**(E5) – Using a visual timetable**
**(E6) – Understanding the concept of 'wait' and using a wait card**
**(E7) – Using visuals to support independence in everyday activities**

*Activity:* Think of a child with ASD who would benefit from one of the visual supports outlined here (E1)–(E7). Plan how you would implement the resource into your setting.

Consider the following:

- In what way will this support the child?
- What will be different after introducing the support; that is, what positive behaviours would you like to see as a result of the visual support being introduced?
- How will you put the strategy in place?
- How you will ensure consistency?

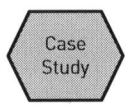

*Case Study:* Alex is three and a half; he has a diagnosis of ASD. He is able to understand short instructions and communicates using short sentences. He loves playing with trains and doesn't want to do anything else at nursery. Recently staff working with him have noticed that he has started to be interested in the sand area when his trains are not visible. Alex can become upset when trains are finished and when he needs to transition onto any other activity.

Table 2.1 Strategy planning sheet: example

| Child's name: | Alex |
|---|---|
| **Strategy/activity to be introduced:** | Using a first/then board (E3) |
| | Understanding the concept 'finished' and using a countdown (E4) |
| **How will this help:** | The first/then board will help Alex understand what is happening next and transition between activities. Staff will encourage Alex to engage in a different activity with trains as a reward, e.g., first sand then trains. |
| **What will be different for Alex:** | He will expand his interests by starting to engage in the sand. |
| | He will become less stressed at transition times as, although it is still a difficult area, he will have had a clear verbal and visual warning when the activity is due to end. |
| **How to implement:** | • Strategy to be discussed at staff meeting |
| | • Strategy planning sheet to be shared with staff (Appendix Two) |
| | • A target sheet (Appendix Three) to be displayed in nursery so all staff are able to implement consistently |

See the Appendix Two planning sheet to photocopy and use this as a template.

Staff working with Alex would like him to engage in other activities and to transition between activities with less upset; they have identified that he will benefit from the use of a first/then board (E3) and countdown (E4).

To ensure that the strategy is implemented effectively, staff have used a planning sheet (Appendix Two) and have paid attention to the steps in Table 2.1.

## Use of routines

We can effectively use routines to help children understand their environment. Many parents of children with ASD tell me that their children learn well through routines. Really, when you think about it, we all learn well, especially when it is new information, in a routine and predictable way. Routines and consistency can make it easier for children with ASD to understand what is happening throughout the day. This can in turn help reduce anxiety. Routines can be comforting for children with ASD and supportive to learning. We can build visual supports, consistent language,

# The early years environment

and songs into our everyday routines to make them more predictable for children with ASD.

- The great thing about routines is that they happen throughout the day so can be a natural way to build in consistent language and learning opportunities.
- You can support a child's understanding in everyday routine activities like hand washing or getting ready for lunch or nap time; this has the added advantage of not feeling like you have to make 'separate time' to work on communication targets.
- Building these key strategies into your routines can have a big impact on the children who you are working with.
- I am often so impressed with the families I work with who take simple strategies and incorporate them into routine activities across the day. This then becomes part of the routine so that the strategies you are using just become automatic.
- Turn now to activity sheet (E8) language for routines for strategies that you can incorporate into your everyday routines.

Let's look at Jack to see how staff working with him used routines and visuals to help him overcome some of the challenges facing him in the environment. His case study is described as follows.

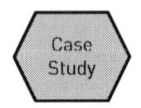

### Case study: supporting Jack's understanding

**Background**

Jack started nursery age two and a half; at this time he was non-verbal with little response to any spoken language. When he started nursery he became upset whenever an adult attempted to direct him onto an activity or take him to change his nappy or wash his hands and would only engage with cars lying down watching them at eye level. He didn't participate in the routines of the nursery and was self-directed. Staff working with him were keen to help him engage more so that he could access new and different learning opportunities.

Jack was unable to ask for anything and would communicate by screaming and pushing items away. He occasionally took an adult's hand to lead to the area he wanted something and would reach towards a preferred item. Often Jack would climb to reach what he wanted and became frustrated when unable to communicate.

### Actions

Staff got to know Jack and completed the Information-Gathering Tool (I-1) and Skills Profile (I-2) several times. From this they were able to identify his profile of strengths and needs. Staff met with Jack's parents to discuss targets. Parents and staff agreed on the following targets (to support understanding):

### Targets

- For Jack to understand the routine of the nursery
- For Jack to understand the concept finished

### Strategies used

Over Jack's first six months staff used the following strategies:

- They consistently used objects to support his understanding (see E1).
- As a staff group they focussed on using consistent language – as outlined in (E8). At a staff meeting they discussed this and realised how much inconsistency there was between them, for example, some people saying 'time for toilet', others saying 'nappy time', and so on.
- They consistently used strategies around helping Jack understand the concept of 'finished' (see E4).
- This particular group of staff were quite musical and decided to introduce a routine song for different activities including tidy up, snack time, shoes on/off, as well as showing an object to support understanding.

### The results

Jack has shown improvements in his understanding. He is now able to respond to cues; for example, when shown a nappy he will now walk towards the change station, and when shown the object for outside he will walk towards the door. One of the major benefits is that he is calm and not becoming distressed with such frequency. Jack plays much less with the cars and now engages with a wider range of activities. Jack has started to hum the tidy-up song at home.

*We will revisit Jack in Chapter Three to look at how staff targeted his expressive communication.*

# The early years environment

## Overcoming challenges by structuring the environment

### Why use structure?

Using structure also supports a child with ASD's strengths; increased structure within the environment provides predictability and reduces confusion. It can promote independence, understanding, and communication and reduce anxiety.

Often when we talk about structure and specifically 'structured teaching', it is in relation to the TEACCH® approach.

### The TEACCH approach

TEACCH® stands for 'Treatment and Education of Autistic and Communication – Handicapped Children'. The approach focusses on the 'culture of autism' as part of its key philosophy. This emphasises the unique strengths and needs of individuals with ASD and considers how the environment and everyday activities need to be adapted to meet these needs.

For more information about TEACCH® see www.teacch.com.

I have attended the TEACCH® training programme twice with Gary Mesibov and found the course truly inspirational.

The TEACCH® approach can be used with people with ASD for all ages and stages from infants to adults. The approach is often used alongside many other approaches. If you are familiar with special schools or specialist resource bases, often the environment is set up in a particular way with workstations for each student. Much of this draws upon the TEACCH® approach.

The TEACCH® programme is based in the University of North Carolina and is used across the whole state of North Carolina and worldwide for infants and adults with ASD. In North Carolina even adults with severe ASD have the opportunity to engage in work. The use of structure and systems enables those with even the most significant needs to carry out activities independently. I remember when completing TEACCH® training watching a film of an adult, with what would be classified as 'severe ASD', working purposefully; this man was competently washing up with the help of several clearly labeled boxes for dirty and clean in addition to tape on the floor showing him where to stand. Such a simple system enables someone with ASD to complete tasks independently and gain the psychological benefit of working.

The TEACCH® approach has five key elements which are useful to be aware of:

- **Physical structure** – This relates to the structure in place within the child or young person's actual environment; this could be the classroom or your home. We all benefit from physical structure in the environment to help us feel organised and understand what is happening, for example, a line on the train platform to show where we need to stand behind. For people with ASD, physical structure gives meaning to the environment through increasing predictability, and makes the environment more organised. The use of structure can support a child or young person's understanding of what is expected in that environment.

- **Visual schedules or timetables** – Schedules, or as they are often known, visual timetables, are a visual representation of what is happening during the day, for example, the morning routine of nursery. Visual timetables can be pictures, written or objects, according to the individual's level of symbolic understanding. Visual timetables aim to increase predictability, help a child understand when changes are going to happen, encourage independence, and reduce anxiety.

- **Activity systems** – In our daily lives we all use lists of what we need to do as part of certain tasks. People with ASD benefit from tasks being presented in a visual way to show what needs to be done and in what order; this is referred to as the activity or work system. As part of this, the student is shown how much work needs to be completed, the sequence the work needs to carried out in, and when the work is finished, and shows the child or young person what they need to do next.

- **Structured activities/tasks** – Within structured activities there is no need for verbal instruction as the visual structure provides a clear outline of the task so that the child is able to complete tasks independently without verbal prompting. The aim is to increase independence and participation.

- **Strengths and interests** – Incorporating a person with ASD's strengths and interests is a key part of the approach; there is an emphasis on using interests to help children engage in other activities. For example, using favourite characters as part of a schedule to increase motivation to engage with it. The world can be a confusing place for children with ASD. Imagine yourself in a totally different country; perhaps everyone is speaking a different language and you can't read the signs or understand what is happening. You don't understand the culture of the place you are in and are not sure where you are meant to be going and what you are meant to be doing. You feel lost and confused.

Then you find yourself a map, start understanding a few key words, and everything starts to make a bit more sense. Phew! You start to relax a little. Perhaps it is not so stressful after all. In the same way as you finding your map and understanding what was going on, we can add structure to make the environment easier to understand and more predictable. This means that children can do the following:

- Understand what we want them to do
- Have less anxiety – remember confusion can lead to anxiety
- Learn independence – we can use structure to help a child learn and carry out tasks independently

Turn now to activity sheets (E9)–(E13), which provide strategies and activities to increase the structure in your environment.

**(E9) – Structuring the learning environment – let's make a plan**
**(E10) – Structuring the learning environment – top tips**
**(E11) – Structuring a one-on-one area using a workstation**
**(E12) – Structuring one-on-one activities**
**(E13) - Managing changes in the routine**

Activity    Complete the planning sheet as part of (E9).

Are there any other ways you can increase structure for the children with ASD who you work with?

Use Appendix Two to plan out implementation of any activities or strategies in the environment.

*The early years environment*

## Environment activity sheet 1. Using objects to support understanding

E:1

**Familiar objects can be used successfully with children with ASD as cues to help their understanding. This may be understanding of what is happening next, who is coming, where they are going, and so on. This can help reduce anxiety and increase predictability of the routine as well as helping children learn to understand the word. Objects used to support understanding in this way are often referred to as 'objects of reference'. Adults working with a child with ASD using 'objects of reference' would typically have a bag of meaningful objects for the child that they would show to support understanding of the routine. Objects can represent people, activities, different times of the day, and places.**

## How to use objects

- Start off by thinking of the routine of the day and which parts would be useful to have an object represent it, for example:
    - Circle time
    - Nappy change/toilet time
    - Outside play
    - Snack/lunch
    - Parent
    - Key worker

- Talk to parents to see which objects you can overlap on. Consistency between home and school is key to supporting understanding.

- Think about the properties of the object as it can be helpful for there to be visual and tactile information as part of the object. For some children tactile information is more meaningful, and a piece of blanket stuck to a small board may be a useful way to signify naptime rather than a soft toy.

- When introducing objects, it is important to consider whether the item is meaningful and relevant for the child; for example, choosing a ball to represent outside play for a child who is not interested in balls will not signify 'outside' in a relevant way.

## When to use objects

- Use objects before the activity is going to happen to support understanding, show the object, and say the word; for example, every time before snack, show a spoon and say 'snack time'.

## How to step it up

If you feel that a child confidently understands objects, it may be worth introducing photos and pictures alongside these with the aim to transition to just photos or pictures. The ability to do this depends on a child's symbolic representation and how easily they understand that a picture, miniature, or object relates to the activity. See the hierarchy of symbolic representation (page 47).

## Materials needed

- Meaningful objects for the child
- Bag to store them

*The early years environment*

## Environment activity sheet 2. Using photos to help understanding

**E:2**

Photos and/or symbols are used widely with children with ASD. As highlighted in Chapter Two, children with ASD are visual learners, so this plays to their strengths. We talk about using photos and pictures across a range of activity sheets in this manual.

As well as supporting understanding, pictures are also often used to help a child's expressive communication; see activity sheet (C9).

Ensure that a child has the symbolic understanding before choosing to use photographs and pictures. Remember that clear photos are easier to understand than abstract symbols.

## How do photos help?

- Unlike a spoken word, which disappears, a picture provides a permanent representation and builds on the philosophy of *'show me, don't tell me'*.

- Using photographs and pictures may be implemented as part of a wider target of using a first/then board or a visual timetable – (E3) and (E5).

- You can use photographs and symbols to offer a cue that is not verbal; this means that instead of always having to tell a child what to do, you can remind them by gently showing a picture; for example, instead of always telling a child to sit still, you could show them a picture of them sitting nicely alongside an 'I am working for' board (B4).

## When to use photographs

- Photographs and pictures are helpful at any time during the day as part of the routine. They can be especially important at transition times or as part of a first/then board or visual timetable.

- Photographs can also be used to reinforce positive behaviours.

- Sometimes when we first introduce photos or pictures, it can be helpful for staff members to wear a lanyard with the symbols easily accessible on it.

# The early years environment

## How to step it up

- As the child becomes accustomed to photographs, you could use them as part of a first/then board or visual timetable.
- As children get older and particularly if they have an interest in letters, make sure that you have the written words alongside the photograph.

## Materials needed

- Photographs
- Laminator

## Environment activity sheet 3. Using a first/then board

E:3

A first/then board presents what we need to do now (first) and what we will do next (then) in a visual way. The board could be a laminated piece of card with attached pictures on or simply a whiteboard or piece of paper with the objects drawn or written on it. You can photocopy the first/then board on page 61 to use in your setting.

### What is a first/then board for?

The first/then board helps children understand the sequence of activities, for example, first story then bubbles. Introducing a first/then board can help with a number of areas including the following:

- Moving a child's attention between activities and understanding when things are finished – you can use the first/then board in conjunction with the strategies outlined on (E4) around finishing activities

- Using the language first/then to help children with sequencing and understanding what's next

- Completing a less-preferred activity when there is a motivating activity next, for example, first wash hands then snack

### How to use a first/then board

- Start off by using it with two activities that the child likes, for example, first bubbles then ball.

- Keep your language simple: 'First bubbles then ball'.

- When the first activity is finished, use a one-minute warning and countdown – five, four, three, two, one – bubbles are finished (with gesture), remove the picture, then show the next one.

- Gradually extend to use the preferred activity second to encourage completion of the first activity.

## The early years environment

**When to use the board:** You can use the first next board throughout the day, but it can be especially helpful at transition times.

## How to step it up

A first/then board (see Figure 2.1) can be a tool to help children move onto using a longer timetable or first/then/then as part of a structured activity. Sharing this strategy with parents can be extremely helpful if they don't already use one. Many parents I have worked with have fed back that using a finished countdown and first/then board has had a significant impact on the number of meltdowns their child has and makes situations like leaving the park much easier.

## Materials needed

- First/then board (template for you to copy and use on the next page) and photos or symbols
- Whiteboard and pens as an alternative

# First/then board

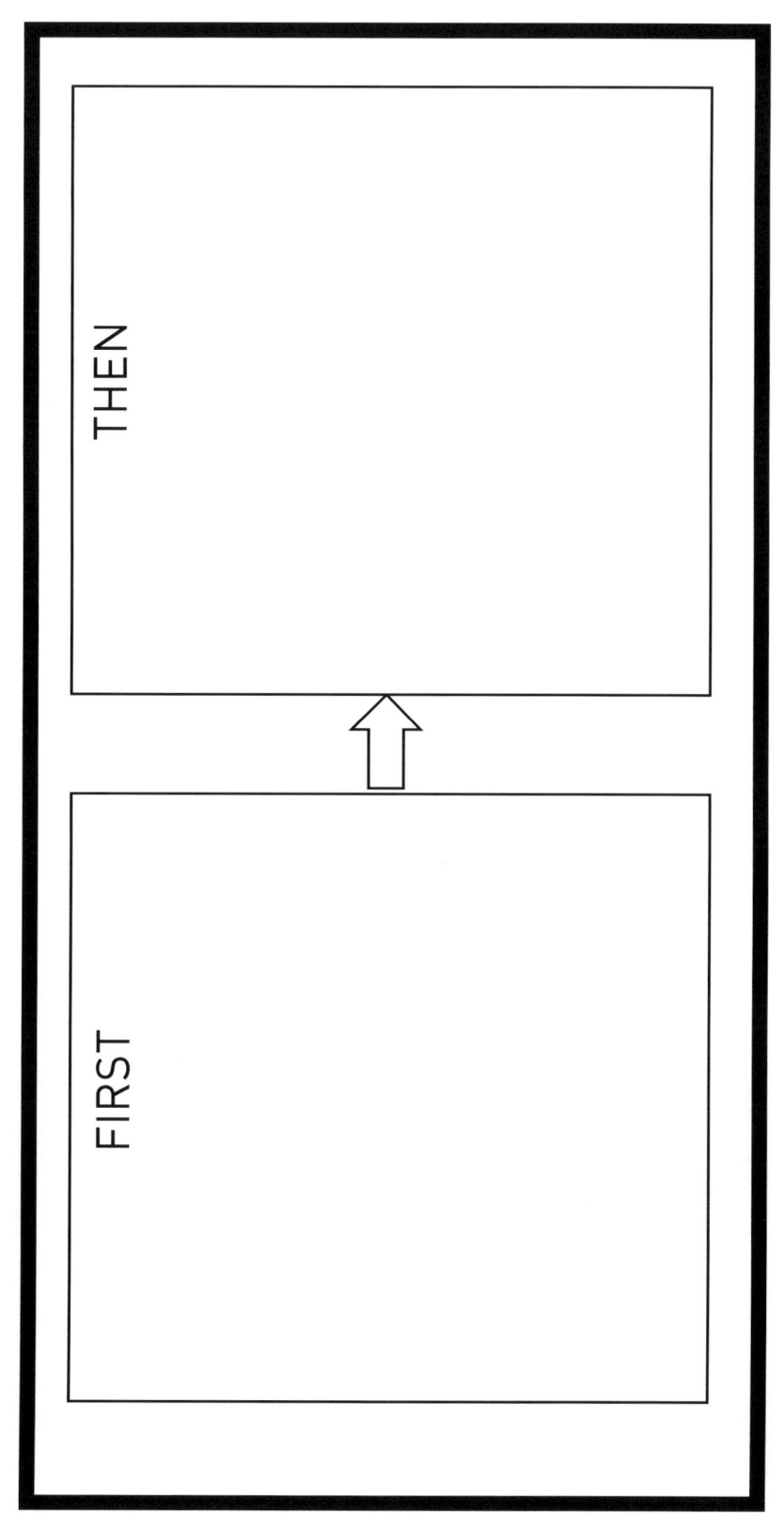

THEN

FIRST

Figure 2.1

*The early years environment*

## Environment activity sheet 4. Understanding the concept 'finished' and using a countdown

**E:4**

Think of all the times in the day that an activity comes to an end and another one starts. A frequent challenge often observed in children with ASD is difficulty around understanding when something has finished and it is time to move onto something new. A first/then board definitely helps with this, but it is helpful to teach children the words and actions associated with 'finished'. I have also noticed that even children who appear to have severe communication difficulties are able to understand this with consistent prompts and use. This can then have quite a profound impact on the child, their parents, and educators by reducing the stress around transitions.

This relates to the 'show me and tell me' idea as often, when a child is busy playing and the adult is telling them it is time to finish, they haven't heard or engaged with the message at all.

## How to teach 'finished'

1 Get down to the child's level, say his or her name, and show your finger indicating one minute: *'Jack, one minute with cars'*. Repeat several times.

2 Still at their level say, 'five, four, three, two, one (whilst showing your fingers, counting down), finished'. When you say 'finished', use a clear hand gesture. Say 'cars have finished' whilst placing the cars into a finished box or bag.

3 Say it is time for blocks (and present next activity).

- **Be consistent** – It is extremely helpful if every member of staff can use a consistent routine (same words and actions) to communicate when an activity is finished. Consistency will help a child understand much quicker.

- **What's next** – It is important for the child to know what is happening next rather than finishing and having nothing to move onto. Often parents and educators say, *'Oh, he is really struggling to finish an activity'*. Think of yourself if you finish something you like doing; it is good to have something else to do. Similarly for the child, remember to show them what they can do next; for example, bubbles have finished, and it is time for books.

## When to use 'finished'

- Use 'finished' at the end of the activity.

- Using a countdown for 'finished' will gradually become incorporated into your use of a first/then board and visual timetable. You will find that it is a useful tool to use in many situations.

## Materials needed

- 'Finished' bag or box

The early years environment

## Environment activity sheet 5. Using a visual timetable

**E:5**

**A visual timetable is a structured way to represent the daily routine in a visual format. The use of a visual timetable can help increase independence, increase predictability, and through this reduce uncertainty and anxiety. A visual timetable helps children understand what is happening next. Using a visual timetable plays to the child with ASD's visual strengths. In many ways we all use something a bit like a visual timetable to help structure our lives, such as a recipe book, a to-do list, or a shopping list. Visual timetables are relevant for all children with ASD, whatever their level of communication; we need to alter how we present the information to them. I have often heard people say that a particular child doesn't need a timetable, only later to wonder why they are struggling when it is time to finish or transition. Visual timetables don't have to be pictures.**

A visual timetable can be made up of the following:

- Objects
- Photographs
- Symbols
- Words

It could be drawn on a whiteboard. It can be organised horizontally or vertically, and it can represent a whole day or a shorter section of time (see Figure 2.2).

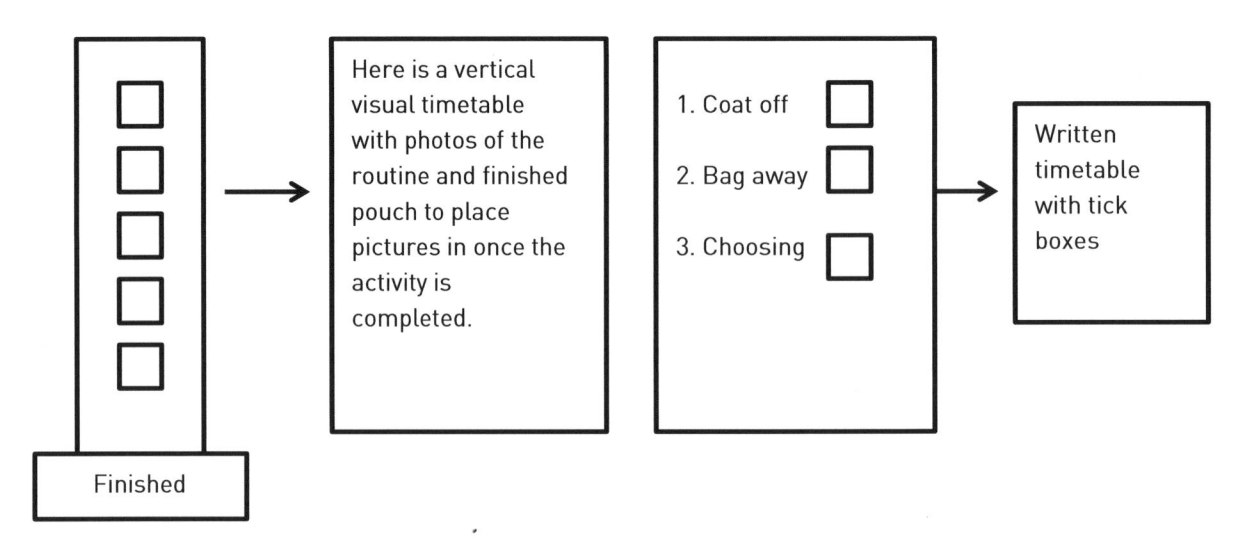

Here is a vertical visual timetable with photos of the routine and finished pouch to place pictures in once the activity is completed.

1. Coat off
2. Bag away
3. Choosing

Written timetable with tick boxes

Finished

Figure 2.2

When setting up a visual timetable you need to consider the following:

- What is the child's level of symbolic understanding?
- How will your organise the pictures?
- Is it the timetable for the whole class or for a particular child?
- How will the child interact with the time table, for example, ticking off each activity, taking it off the picture strip, and placing it in the 'finished' box?

## Materials needed

- Photos or symbols
- Whiteboard

The early years environment

**Environment activity sheet 6.
Understanding the concept of 'wait' and
using a wait card**

E:6

'Waiting' is a difficult concept to understand. All children regardless of having SEND or SLCN can find waiting difficult. In my experience it can be a challenge for children with ASD that parents and educators frequently want to address. Not being able to wait can be stressful to both children and those working with them. This can also have a big impact on parents' lives; when children are struggling to wait for a bus or in the shopping queue, this can be stressful for the child. The tricky thing about waiting is that it is quite an abstract concept. You can't see 'wait' in the same way you can 'drink' or 'snack'. We need to be creative to think about how we can make the concept 'wait' more concrete.

### Teach 'waiting' at the right time

- Often we are asking children to wait at a time when they are already finding it difficult as in they are already not waiting; e.g., we are saying, 'Wait, wait', whilst they are trying to push their way in front of another child in the queue for the slide.

- We need to start commenting on when children are waiting in positive situations, for example, waiting for a snack or waiting at the traffic lights.

- We can focus specifically on 'waiting' to teach it in games and positive activities.

### Top tips

- Make it visual. Use a consistent gesture to accompany your words.

- Use a wait card. This is typically a card like the one that follows (with a coloured background). Every time children are waiting, show them the card as a prompt. Use consistent language, for example, 'Waiting' or 'You are waiting'.

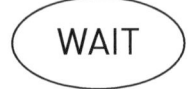

( WAIT )

- How long am I waiting for? Sand timers and countdown timers also have the benefit of showing a child how long they need to wait.

- Consider how long you expect a child to wait. Be realistic; start with a short time and gradually increase it.

# The early years environment

- Tell the children what is happening after they are waiting; this may be clear, but you could provide a visual reminder, for example, with a first/then board (E3) or by using photographs to support understanding (E4), for example, 'waiting for snack'.
- Remember to say what is happening in the order that it is happening.
- Give specific praise to reinforce positive behaviour. (See Chapter Six.)

## Materials needed

- Wait card

*The early years environment*

## Environment activity sheet 7. Using visuals to support independence in everyday activities

E:7

**We know from reading Chapter Two that using visuals can help children be more independent. Knowing what happens next can reduce anxiety and increase confidence along with a range of other skills.**

**We can use visuals to support independence in everyday activities; these work well in conjunction with the home setting.**

A timetable, as described in (E5), can be used to break down everyday activities. Visuals are commonly used as part of the following everyday sequences:

- Toileting
- Getting dressed
- Leaving and getting to the nursery
- Bedtime routine
- Morning routine

It may be that at the end of the sequence, there is a reward shown to motivate the child through the sequence, for example:

- Breakfast
- Clothes on
- Clean teeth
- Shoes on
- Five minutes of TV

As with (E5) this could be on a vertical or a horizontal timetable either in a fixed point or on a strip that the child carries around. Don't worry if you don't have the individual symbols or pictures to hand. Draw the routine out on the whiteboard.

*Activity:* Think of a child in your setting; is there a routine or activity that he or she could work towards completing independently with visual supports?

Many parents spend a lot of time working on independence at home; working collaboratively on these areas will be supportive. Toileting or dressing (if the child is developmentally ready) can be great shared goals to target. The use of visual support can be helpful to show the child what the expectation is.

## Materials needed

- Photographs or symbols
- Whiteboard and pens

*The early years environment*

## Environment activity sheet 8. Language for routines

**E:8**

Adding language to routines and activities can be a powerful strategy to help children develop understanding of language. Using consistent words and phrases at certain times of the day and in certain activities also provides children with a model of what they need to say and do. Routines are consistent, which then allows for regular opportunities for children to hear the same words, which allows for language learning.

One of the most powerful, easy-to-use strategies to enable children to understand us is to use less language when you are talking. Often we don't realise that we are using long sentences, which makes it hard for a child to understand or latch onto the particular word as part of the routine.

### Language is not just talking

Adding gestures and pointing is another visual way of helping a child understand the words and environment.

### Top tips for adding language to routines

- Use less language.
- Repeat key words and phrases.
- Talk about what the child is doing – this helps children learn action words.
- Add gestures.
- Be consistent.
- Be musical and creative, for example, singing a tidy-up song or hello or good-bye song every day. Routine songs can be helpful in helping a child understand the routine.
- Use the child's interests.

For a child with limited understanding, instead of saying, 'Let's go and wash hands now; our hands are all dirty', try pointing at the dirty hands, saying 'dirty', then pointing to the sink and saying 'wash hands' (whilst using a gesture and using a visual support). To begin with it can feel quite unnatural to be saying less; think of it as communicating at the right level for the child.

## Materials needed

- None

*The early years environment*

## Environment activity sheet 9. Structuring the learning environment – let's make a plan

**E:9**

Earlier in chapter we discussed the TEACCH® approach and one of the key principles of structuring the environment. Within the TEACCH® programme this is referred to as the 'physical structure' and refers to the actual surroundings and arrangement of the person with ASD's learning or home environment. We can structure the environment to include different areas for work, snack, play, calming area, books, or whichever areas that are specific to your environment.

**We know that structure can help to accomplish the following:**

- **Reduce anxiety**
- **Increase understanding**
- **Promote independence**

## Planning the environment?

Learning environments often have quite clear boundaries in terms of different areas, for example, home corner, snack area, toilet, and hand washing. These clearly defined 'zoned' areas can be helpful for children with ASD.

The aim in planning the environment is to think about whether we can make any of the areas any clearer in terms of their function.

- Turn to the planning sheet on the following page, which can be photocopied.
- Draw out your learning space.
- Label the different areas.
- From your plan is it clear what each area is for?
- What areas already have a clear structure, and what areas could be clearer? Use the planning sheet to think about your space.
- Is there any furniture you could use to create clearer 'zones' (e.g., instead of having a bookcase against the wall, turn it to create a clearer reading corner)?
- Think about how you can label the areas using visual supports.

**Activity** Draw your space below – clearly label different areas.

Copyright material from Jennifer Warwick (2020) *Supporting SLCN in Children with ASD in the Early Years*, Routledge

*The early years environment*

## Environment activity sheet 10.
## Structuring the learning environment – top tips

**E:10**

**We know that adding structure to the learning environment is a positive strategy for children with ASD. This is a key feature of the TEACCH® approach.**

**Now that you have completed your plan (E8), think about which areas in your learning environment you can bring more structure to.**

(Activity) Brainstorm how you can bring more structure to your environment.

Add your ideas to (E9). The ideas that follow may be relevant to your setting.

### Boundaries

It may feel that the areas of the classroom are clearly defined; think about it from the perspective of a child with ASD. Would it make sense? Could you add any physical markers, for example, masking tape on the floor, or position the furniture in a certain way so that each area is clearly defined?

### Lining up

Using tape on the floor to make a line to show children where to stand can be a helpful and simple way to add structure to the environment. You could also use a visual support to indicate who is going to go first in the line and also a wait card (E6).

### Circle time

Using a carpet spot or square or even a sticker on the floor, if the others are too distracting, can be a clear way to show a child where he or she needs to sit.

### Colours

Using different-colour tables and chairs or even adding a different colour tablecloth can be a helpful way of creating different 'zones' in the environment. This is also a helpful way of helping a child understand different activities in the same space; for example, a yellow table covering could indicate snack, and blue could indicate messy play.

## Quiet area

Having a clear 'quiet area' can be helpful for all children within the environment. Zone a quiet area for children with beanbags or even a tent. Within this quiet area, consider the amount of information on display. It may be that you choose neutral colours without decoration on the walls within this area so that it is less visually stimulating. I once worked in a special school for children with ASD where all the classroom walls were blue and there were minimal visual distractions, particularly in the quiet or calm area; it made a real difference.

## Outside play

Outside play naturally lends itself to having clearly defined different areas: for example, messy sand and water, a pretend play area with a toy house, and physical play. If you have bikes or equipment that requires children to take turns, consider using a timer or turn-taking board (S8).

## Materials needed

- Based on your planning outlined in (E9)

The early years environment

## Environment activity sheet 11.
## Structuring a one-on-one area using a workstation

E:11

**A workstation is a key part of the structured teaching method outlined as part of the TEACCH® approach. Like much of the TEACCH® philosophy, using a workstation incorporates routine, visual cues, routine, and structure as well as limiting distractions. Use of a workstation aims to help children with ASD develop independence and organisational skills. Workstations can be helpful for one-on-one work where you need a child to work independently on tasks. If your local area has an ASD outreach service, this may be something that a teacher is able to support you with. This activity sheet provides a brief overview.**

The workstation shows a child these steps:

- What I need to do

- How much work there is to do

- How do I know that I have finished

- What happens next

In my experience workstations are often used incorrectly. Instead of focussing on activities that children can complete independently, they become one-on-one teaching areas. A workstation should focus on activities the child can do with a focus on independence. You can offer an occasional physical prompt, but do not give verbal instructions. Limit any verbal prompts (see Figure 2.3).

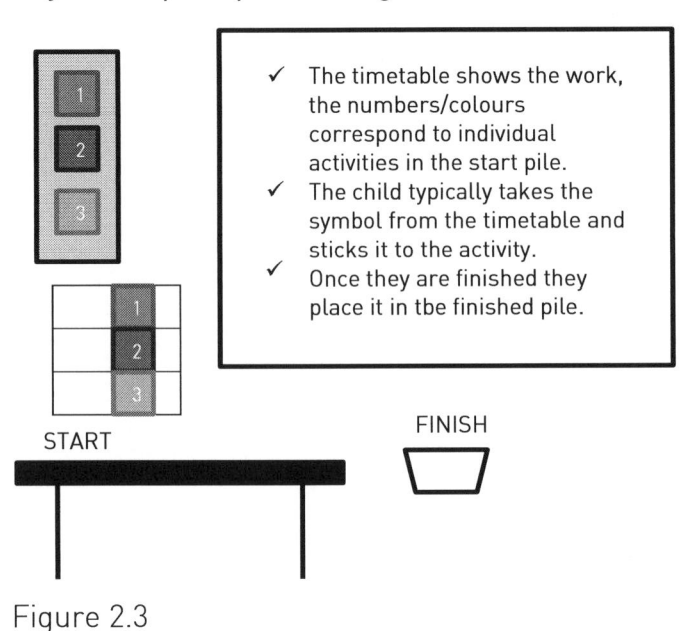

✓ The timetable shows the work, the numbers/colours correspond to individual activities in the start pile.
✓ The child typically takes the symbol from the timetable and sticks it to the activity.
✓ Once they are finished they place it in tbe finished pile.

START    FINISH

Figure 2.3

## What activities to use

- Use activities that the children are competent in so they are able to carry them out independently.
- Puzzles and manipulation tasks work well.
- Shoebox tasks, available to purchase, can work well.
- Any activity can be adapted to be a workstation activity.

## Materials needed

- Table
- Plastic trays
- Plastic wallets for activities

## The early years environment

### Environment activity sheet 12. Structuring one-on-one activities

**E:12**

We can use structure and visual support to enable a child to be more independent within an activity. This is particularly helpful for children who are prompt, dependent, and reliant on an adult to tell them what to do every step of the way.

Basically, this is like a visual timetable for within the activity. It breaks the activity down to show the child each component part. This is easily adapted to many activities and can be used in conjunction with other children as part of a small group or at the workstation.

Using visual supports like these in activities is helpful for children with English as an additional language and all SLCN.

The following example breaks down a short craft activity.

### Making a sparkly heart

As with the first/then board, you could draw the sequence out on a small whiteboard. This has the advantage that it is quick and portable, and you can quickly get in the habit of using it to break down many activities (see Figure 2.4).

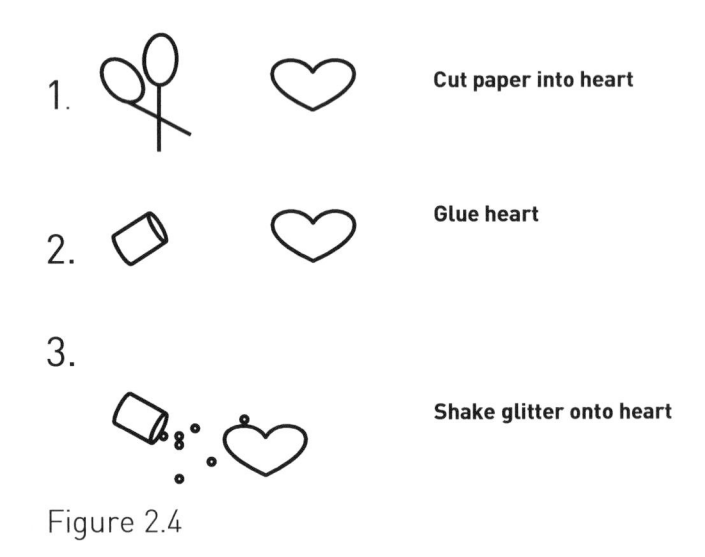

1. **Cut paper into heart**

2. **Glue heart**

3. **Shake glitter onto heart**

Figure 2.4

### Materials needed

- Whiteboard
- Whiteboard pens

# The early years environment

## Environment activity sheet 13. Managing changes in the routine

**E:13**

**We can support a child's understanding of the routine using a visual timetable which can help significantly. Sometimes there are unexpected changes to the routine, for example, a trip out with the education environment or a change to the usual activities such as a Christmas play. It is important that children with ASD are able to learn how to accept changes to the routine.**

**We can support children's understanding of these changes by using the following strategies.**

## Preparation

- Use visual supports to help prepare a child. For example, for a trip have an individual timetable of the day's routine including mode of transpiration, activities, and what is happening at the end. Take a whiteboard as backup.

- If it is a school trip, parents could visit with the child before. I worked once with a child who started doing this for the first few visits. His family visited the place (a museum in Central London) at the weekend and took a series of photos, which were then printed out and added to a social story (Gray, 2019). This prepared the child effectively and significantly reduced anxiety before the trip.

- You can prepare children for new experiences; for example, if they have never been to a birthday party, you can use a short social story (Gray, 2019) about birthday parties and what to expect. This has the advantage of reinforcing positive social behaviours.

## Teach flexibility

- We know that children with ASD like routine and predictability. We can use these strategies to help teach children to be flexible. For example, have a calendar and talk about days that are different in advance, for example, Christmas, Halloween, and class trips.

- Use a surprise symbol on the visual timetable to indicate that something different may be happening.

# The early years environment

> **Chapter Two summary**
>
> - The education environment and early years curriculum can be stressful and overwhelming for a child with ASD.
>
> - We can make positive changes to the environment to make it more predictable for children with ASD.
>
> - We can use a child with ASD's strength in visual processing and introduce a range of visual supports depending on their level of symbolic representation.
>
> - Increasing structure as part of the routine helps increase the child's understanding of the environment.
>
> - Activity sheets (E1)–(E13) all provide practical tips on how to support understanding and making the learning environment more accessible for children with ASD.

## References

Gray, C. (2019). *Carol Gray Social Stories*. https://carolgraysocialstories.com/.

Mesibov, G. B. and Shea, V. (2010). The TEACCH® program in the era of evidence-based practice. *Journal of Autism and Developmental Disorders*, 40(5), 570–579.

# Chapter Three
# COMMUNICATION SKILLS

**Chapter Three provides the following:**

- An overview of communication development in typical children and children with ASD
- A summary of joint attention
- Practical case studies to illustrate the communication needs of children with ASD
- Activity sheets:

    **(C1) – Developing joint and shared attention**

    **(C2) – The power of pausing**

    **(C3) – Imitation 'copy me'!**

    **(C4) – Making chances to communicate – offering choices**

    **(C5) – Making chances to communicate – giving**

    **(C6) – Making chances to communicate – a bit at a time**

    **(C7) – Ready, steady, go games**

    **(C8) – Stop/go games**

    **(C9) – Making choices with a choosing board**

    (C10) – Asking for help

    (C11) – Using songs

    (C12) – Adding language

    (C13) – Using action words

    (C14) – Reducing repeated language

    (C15) – Let's create

    (C16) – Using an about-me book

# Communication skills

## Development of communication

Communication develops even before a child is born; in the womb babies are becoming familiar with the native language spoken in their environment. From soon after birth babies develop their sociocognitive skills, receptive language (understanding), and expressive language (spoken language). Typically, children start to understand words before they are able to say them. Even before children are talking, they are developing important skills. Receptive and expressive language are self-explanatory, but what do we mean by sociocognitive skills?

Sociocognitive skills relate to basic skills in engaging and interacting with others and are important skills in the development of communication, social interaction, and play. In typically developing children these skills are innate and are crucial to the development of both language and also social communication. These skills include (amongst others) joint and shared attention and social responsiveness in addition to gesture and symbolic understanding. These skills all play a part in two-way communication. Typically children do not need to learn these skills; they just have them. Think of a baby or young child of one year old; typically when you smile at them, they smile at you, or if you look or point to an item out of sight, they are intrigued and interested to know what you are looking at. We are naturally programmed to be social, and from an early age, long before we can talk, we are learning how to use these skills.

We know that communication is so much more than words. Gestures, symbolic understanding, and joint and shared attention all play a huge part in the development of typical communication

The FIRST WORDS PROJECT® is an extremely useful resource for practitioners and parents. They have kindly given permission to use a number of their checklists in this manual. These checklists provide you with a detailed insight of what to expect at different ages and stages.

*Activity* — Read "Milestones That Matter Most" and "16 Gestures by 16 Months" on the next few pages regarding the development of typical communication. These are used with permission from The FIRST WORDS PROJECT® (www.firstwordsproject.com), copyright © 2019 Florida State University. All rights reserved.

Think about what may be different in a child with ASD who has a disordered pattern of communication.

# SOCIAL COMMUNICATION GROWTH CHARTS
## Milestones that Matter Most

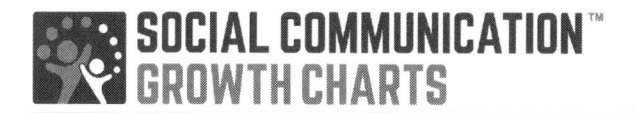

Early communication sets the stage for talking, learning, and later success in life. What you do and say now can make all the difference in your baby's development. Especially because your baby's brain is developing at an amazing rate.

Our Social Communication Milestones cover 5 developmental domains—Play, Language, Social Interaction, Emotional Regulation, and Self-Directed Learning—with two developmental threads in each domain. Here you will find a list of 10 milestones every 2 months. Follow the threads to find out what's in store for your baby from 7 to 24 months and celebrate as your baby reaches each new milestone.

For more detail on our **Social Communication Milestones**, click on your child's age to download and print the milestones every 2 months with lots of examples.

Learn how you can join our **Social Communication Growth Charts**—a powerful new online tool to help parents encourage the milestones that matter most, with videos to explore and questions to chart your child's growth.

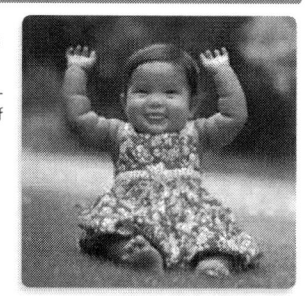

## 7-8 MONTHS

|  |  |  |
|---|---|---|
| Language | Gestures & Meanings | I can use my hands to take things and move my body toward what interests me. |
| | Sounds & Words | I can make different noises with my mouth and different sounds. |
| Play | Using Actions with Objects | I can grasp, hold, bang, mouth, and let go of objects to explore how they work. |
| | Social Sharing with Objects | I am interested in exploring objects with you and noticing your reactions. |
| Social Interaction | Social Attention | I notice you, look at you often, and can easily shift my attention to you when you talk or gesture. |
| | Intentional Communication | I am learning you are the agent of change. |
| Emotional Regulation | Sharing & Managing Emotions | I can smile, laugh, and use my voice when I'm happy. |
| | Regulating Challenging Moments | I can use different actions and sounds, in addition to crying, when I'm upset. |
| Self-Directed Learning | Understanding Messages | I can use different actions and sounds that show I anticipate what will happen next. |
| | Creating New Ideas | I am interested in learning what I can do with objects. |

## 9-10 MONTHS

|  |  |  |
|---|---|---|
| Language | Gestures & Meanings | I can use early gestures like giving and reaching to get you to do something. |
| | Sounds & Words | I can use my voice to make different sounds to let you know how I feel. |
| Play | Using Actions with Objects | I can explore objects and repeat different actions with objects. |
| | Social Sharing with Objects | I enjoy and anticipate your actions. |
| Social Interaction | Social Attention | I notice you and what you're looking at. |
| | Intentional Communication | I can let you know what I want and what I don't want. |
| Emotional Regulation | Sharing & Managing Emotions | I can share happy moments when I interact with you. |
| | Regulating Challenging Moments | I can share sad or frustrated feelings to get you to comfort me. |
| Self-Directed Learning | Understanding Messages | I can guess what you're about to do and use "hints" around me to understand your message. |
| | Creating New Ideas | I notice you and listen to your voice to guide my actions. |

## 11-12 MONTHS

|  |  |  |
|---|---|---|
| Language | Gestures & Meanings | I can use gestures like showing and pointing to get you to notice what I am interested in. |
| | Sounds & Words | I can use speech sounds together as if I am "talking" to you. |
| Play | Using Actions with Objects | I can use functional actions with several objects. |
| | Social Sharing with Objects | I enjoy taking turns exchanging objects with you. |
| Social Interaction | Social Attention | I am eager to interact with you and help keep the interaction going. |
| | Intentional Communication | I can get you to notice me and things I'm interested in. |
| Emotional Regulation | Sharing & Managing Emotions | I can share enjoyment and flow with transitions between activities. |
| | Regulating Challenging Moments | I can hang in there during a necessary activity and do things to make myself feel better. |
| Self-Directed Learning | Understanding Messages | I can follow simple directions like "come here" or "give it to me" when you ask me with gestures. |
| | Creating New Ideas | I watch you and try to do something with you or take on a job I can do with a little help. |

## 13-14 MONTHS

|  |  |  |
|---|---|---|
| Language | Gestures & Meanings | I can learn new gestures like clapping and blowing a kiss by watching and imitating you. |
| | Sounds & Words | I can use a few protowords or early forms of words in familiar situations. |
| Play | Using Actions with Objects | I can use functional actions with you or a stuffed animal. |
| | Social Sharing with Objects | I can learn new actions with objects by watching and imitating you. |
| Social Interaction | Social Attention | I can watch you and imitate what you do and say. |
| | Intentional Communication | I can communicate to share my enjoyment and interests with you. |
| Emotional Regulation | Sharing & Managing Emotions | I can seek out situations that are fun, invite you to join me, and insist on being part of the action. |
| | Regulating Challenging Moments | I can make it clear to you that I do not "want" something or do not want "to do" something. |
| Self-Directed Learning | Understanding Messages | I can listen to you and try to figure out your message. |
| | Creating New Ideas | I can communicate my preference when you offer several choices or let you know I want something else. |

Developed by the FIRST WORDS Project    Copyright © 2019 Florida State University. All rights reserved.

# SOCIAL COMMUNICATION™ GROWTH CHARTS

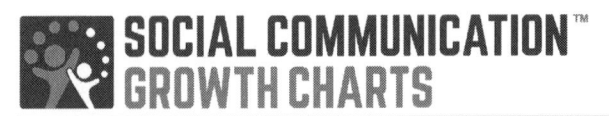

## Milestones that Matter Most

### 15-16 MONTHS

| Category | Subcategory | Milestone |
|---|---|---|
| Language | Gestures & Meanings | I can use symbolic gestures to share ideas with you. |
| Language | Sounds & Words | I can use at least 5 different words that mean something to both of us. |
| Play | Using Actions with Objects | I can use pretend actions with objects that have imagined things from everyday activities. |
| Play | Social Sharing with Objects | I can use objects in a silly, playful way and in a way that helps you get things done. |
| Social Interaction | Social Attention | I can communicate to get your attention and check in with you regularly. |
| Social Interaction | Intentional Communication | I try to figure out what you mean and keep the interaction going. |
| Emotional Regulation | Sharing & Managing Emotions | I can stay active and engaged with you in fun situations and in necessary activities. |
| Emotional Regulation | Regulating Challenging Moments | I can tolerate you helping me stick with a task, even when I am upset. |
| Self-Directed Learning | Understanding Messages | I can respond when you talk to me and share my ideas with you. |
| Self-Directed Learning | Creating New Ideas | I can be productive doing my job and stand my ground with you. |

### 17-18 MONTHS

| Category | Subcategory | Milestone |
|---|---|---|
| Language | Gestures & Meanings | I can look at you and use a gesture and word together to tell you what I am thinking. |
| Language | Sounds & Words | I can use at least 10 different words that mean something to both of us. |
| Play | Using Actions with Objects | I can pretend using new actions that you show me or tell me to do. |
| Play | Social Sharing with Objects | I can use several objects together to build or create something with you. |
| Social Interaction | Social Attention | I can hang in and do something with you and monitor what you're paying attention to. |
| Social Interaction | Intentional Communication | I try to help you know what I mean by adding information to my message. |
| Emotional Regulation | Sharing & Managing Emotions | I can get motivated or settle down with the help of your words and stay available for learning. |
| Emotional Regulation | Regulating Challenging Moments | I can shift attention from something I want to do and engage in a different activity with you. |
| Self-Directed Learning | Understanding Messages | I can understand words without gestures in familiar situations. |
| Self-Directed Learning | Creating New Ideas | I notice opportunities for interaction and learning and can get myself involved. |

### 19-20 MONTHS

| Category | Subcategory | Milestone |
|---|---|---|
| Language | Gestures & Meanings | I can use my words to share something interesting and to protest something I don't want. |
| Language | Sounds & Words | I can use at least 20 words to name people, animals, body parts, objects, actions, and places. |
| Play | Using Actions with Objects | I can pretend using actions with imagined things from less familiar activities. |
| Play | Social Sharing with Objects | I can combine different types of materials to create a play scenario with you. |
| Social Interaction | Social Attention | I am eager to share my interests and ideas with you. |
| Social Interaction | Intentional Communication | I can persist in communicating my message to you. |
| Emotional Regulation | Sharing & Managing Emotions | I can share enjoyment with my words and gestures and stay engaged in the activity with you. |
| Emotional Regulation | Regulating Challenging Moments | I can say or do something that helps me manage my emotions and stay focused in a necessary activity. |
| Self-Directed Learning | Understanding Messages | I can follow simple directions when you ask me to do something. |
| Self-Directed Learning | Creating New Ideas | I can recognize a problem or challenge and try to figure out what to do. |

### 21-22 MONTHS

| Category | Subcategory | Milestone |
|---|---|---|
| Language | Gestures & Meanings | I can learn many new words every week and use them to share ideas with you. |
| Language | Sounds & Words | I can use at least 50 words and combine two words to convey different meanings. |
| Play | Using Actions with Objects | I can combine two different pretend actions with imagined things in a play scenario. |
| Play | Social Sharing with Objects | I can tell you about my play scenario and invite you to play with me. |
| Social Interaction | Social Attention | I can take a few turns sharing my ideas and listening to your ideas. |
| Social Interaction | Intentional Communication | I can ask you about things that I don't know. |
| Emotional Regulation | Sharing & Managing Emotions | I can use my words to ask you to help me get motivated or settle down. |
| Emotional Regulation | Regulating Challenging Moments | My very upset moments are getting briefer and I can flow with unpleasant or unexpected situations. |
| Self-Directed Learning | Understanding Messages | I can observe and listen to you to know what I am supposed to do and go along with your plan. |
| Self-Directed Learning | Creating New Ideas | I can come up a creative idea and let you know my plan. |

### 23-24 MONTHS

| Category | Subcategory | Milestone |
|---|---|---|
| Language | Gestures & Meanings | I can use phrases that describe things and request new information. |
| Language | Sounds & Words | I can use at least 100 words in phrases that include names, actions, and descriptions. |
| Play | Using Actions with Objects | I can combine several different pretend actions in a logical sequence. |
| Play | Social Sharing with Objects | I can begin to take on a make-believe role in a pretend play scenario with you. |
| Social Interaction | Social Attention | I can talk with you about a topic I'm interested in like we're having a conversation. |
| Social Interaction | Intentional Communication | I can let you know how I feel and negotiate when things don't go my way. |
| Emotional Regulation | Sharing & Managing Emotions | I can use my words to share moments of success with you. |
| Emotional Regulation | Regulating Challenging Moments | I can calm myself down, come back to you, and communicate what I want or need. |
| Self-Directed Learning | Understanding Messages | I can create opportunities to learn about things that interest me in everyday situations. |
| Self-Directed Learning | Creating New Ideas | I can try out new things and seek out new opportunities for learning. |

Developed by the FIRST WORDS Project. Copyright © 2019 Florida State University. All rights reserved.

# A Glimpse of our 16 Gestures by 16 Months

**16 by 16**

Research shows the development of gestures predicts language skills 2 years later. Children should be using at least 2 new gestures each month from 9 to 16 months. By 16 months, children should have at least 16 gestures.

**9 Months:** Give, Shake head

**10 Months:** Reach, Raise arms

**11 Months:** Show, Wave

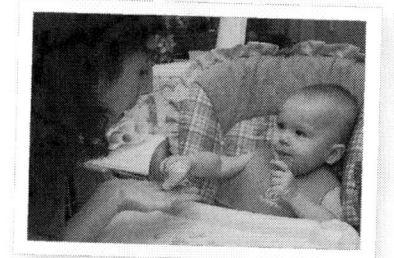

**12 Months:** Open hand, Point, Tap

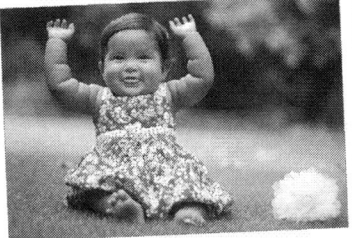

**13 Months:** Clap, Blow a kiss

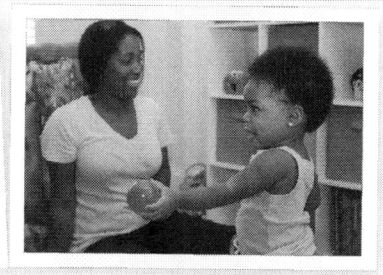

**14 Months:** Index finger point, Shhh gesture

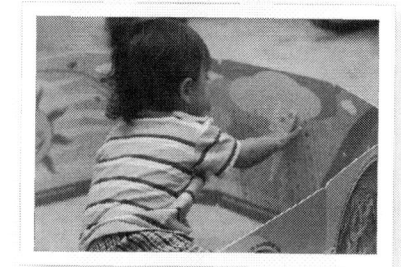

**15 Months:** Head nod, Thumbs up, Hand up

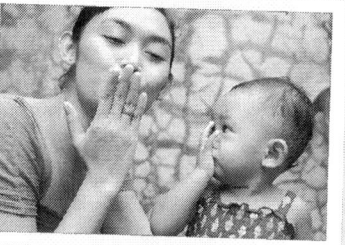

**16 Months:** Other symbolic gestures

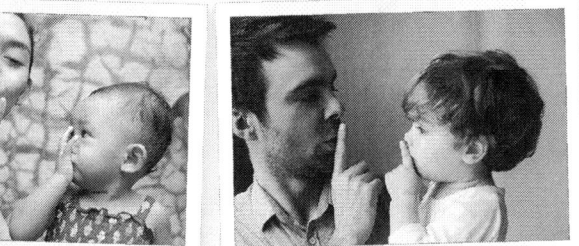

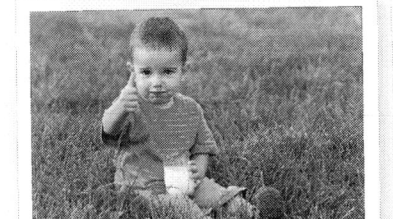

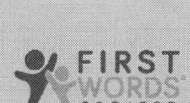

**FIRST WORDS PROJECT**

Visit www.FirstWordsProject.com to print, download, and share the complete 16 Gestures by 16 Months and explore our Lookbook.

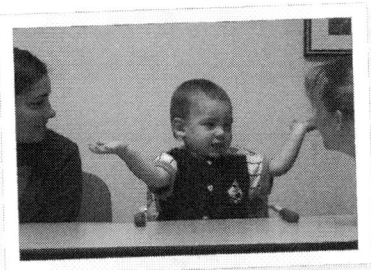

**Screen My Child**

If your child is between 9 and 18 months, we invite you to participate in our research and have your child screened with the Smart ESAC.

*Find out how at*
**FirstWordsProject.com**

*While you are there*

**CHECK OUT OUR GROWTH CHARTS**

Learn the Milestones that Matter Most.

Copyright © 2018 Florida State University. All rights reserved.

# Communication Skills

## Joint attention

SLTs often talk about joint attention as a key part of communication and social interaction development. You will have gained some understanding from reading the checklist and also your reading in Chapter One. We will turn now to consider joint attention and why it is important for communication and social interaction.

## What is joint attention?

Joint attention relates to the ability to share a focus of attention with someone else. Typically, joint attention emerges in young children towards the end of their first year of life and involves both responding to joint attention and initiating joint attention. These skills are important for developing attention, looking and listening to activities together, learning new words, and engaging in interaction with others.

- **Responding to joint attention** – This involves looking and focussing on where someone is looking and/or pointing, for example, when you are walking along with a child and you say, 'Look, bus', whilst looking and pointing towards it. Typically, children will look to where you are pointing and see the bus whilst hearing the word at the same time.

- **Initiating joint attention** – This is being able to get someone else to focus on something of interest, for example, when a child points to an airplane and says, 'Uh uh', whilst looking back at you to make sure you are looking at it as well.

## Why is joint attention so important?

In Chapter One we discussed theory of mind; research indicates that joint attention is an important precursor to the development of theory of mind; it is suggested that at around seven to nine months children start to understand attention and they are also beginning to understand another person's thoughts. In other words, when a young child directs another person's attention by pointing for example to a bus he or she has the ability to consider that another person may find what the bus that he or she is looking at interesting

Joint attention is also important for learning new words and giving meaning to objects. Think of a young, typically developing child, age eighteen months, walking in a buggy with his mother. The bus goes past, and the mother points to the bus and says, 'Look, bus' (whilst pointing). Because the child is able to follow her point and responds immediately to her, he is able to put the big, red, shiny object (bus) and the word 'bus' together. Similarly, later on in the day when walking through the park, the child sees a dog, points, and says, 'Woof'. The mother also points and says, 'Yes, dog'. Without joint and shared attention, it can be much harder for children to learn words in this way.

## Attention and listening versus joint attention

Joint attention is quite an abstract concept and isn't something I regularly see educators attempting to develop. Sometimes there can be confusion between attention and listening skills and joint attention.

Often when I visit nurseries, staff have concerns that a child 'won't pay attention' or 'won't sit at a table or group time'. Naturally there is a tendency to want to develop attention and listening skills as they have such a big impact on all other areas, and this then becomes a goal as part of an individual education plan; for example, 'Jack will sit for 10 minutes at story time'. In many cases a goal like this is asking too much in terms of what they are able to focus on. Whilst all children do need to develop their ability to pay attention to others as part of activities, it is important with children with ASD that this is done in a way that is at the child's level. Often sitting in a circle and listening to a story is not motivating enough for a child with ASD to attend to.

Often the activities that we expect a child to engage in within an early years education environment are at a higher level (level 5–level 6) than their skills are at (level 1–level 4). Table 3.1 outlines the stages of attention and provides some simple strategies for each level. Information regarding the levels of attention adapted from Cooper, Moodley and Reynell (1978).

**Activity** Look at the stages of attention in the Skills Profile or in Table 3.1. Think about a child you work with, and think what level of attention they are at. Think about the activities they can and can't engage with. What is the difference?

Table 3.1 Stages of attention, implications, and support strategies

| Stage of attention | What this looks like | What the impact is | Support strategies |
|---|---|---|---|
| **Level 1** – Very distractible with fleeting attention only | The child's attention is on whatever is their current interest and will be quickly shifted to anything new. | Unable to attend to any adult led tasks. | Find out what is interesting to the child. Follow his or her lead and incorporate these into what you are doing. See (C1) and (C2). |
| **Level 2** – Attends to own choice of activity for a longer period of time but cuts self off from everything else | Can concentrate on a task of their own choosing. A child at this stage does not have the ability to focus on more than one task. It is difficult for an adult to direct the child onto tasks that are not motivating for him or her. | Unable to engage with activities that are not interesting to them. Difficulties with transitions. | Before giving an instruction get down to the child's level and say his or her name. A visual prompt or touching his or her arm will also be a helpful cue. Use a countdown and strategies to support understanding around 'finished' (E4). |
| **Level 3** – Still single-channelled attention but begins to attend to adults | Children at this stage will still focus on self-chosen activities, often for long periods, but they are starting to able to shift their attention between activities with adult support. | Without adult support, will focus only on self-selected activities. Difficulties with transitions. | Gain the child's attention before giving any instructions or expecting a response. Call his or her name before speaking. Use a child's interests to encourage engaging in a wider range of activities (P1). Use a first/then board (E3) and consistent use of countdown (E4) to support understanding of the concept 'finished'. |
| **Level 4** – Still single-channelled but able to shift attention between tasks with prompts | Children at this stage begin to be able to control their own focus of attention. They require less adult support to shift their attention to and from activities more easily. | Difficulties in attending flexibly to tasks. | Use visual prompts, e.g., a visual timetable (E5) and photographs to support understanding (E2). Give information in a clear sequence. Talk about things happening in the order that they occur. |

| Stage of attention | What this looks like | What the impact is | Support strategies |
|---|---|---|---|
| **Level 5** – Integrated attention for short periods of time | Children at this stage has 'dual-channelled attention'; this means that they can be doing something whilst listening to an adult giving instructions. Able to cope with group situations. | Attention can still be quite short at times. | Encourage active listening; give specific praise for good listening. |
| **Level 6** – Integrated attention well established | A child at this stage has flexible attention and is able to sustain focus for lengthy periods of time. The child can integrate visual and auditory information with ease. | | Encourage active questioning and processing of information. |

## Development of communication in children with ASD

Children with ASD develop communication in an atypical way; often SLTs will describe it as following a 'disordered pattern of development'. These means that the communication skills of children with ASD aren't behind their developmental stage and age; they are developing in an uneven way. Even amongst children with ASD of the same age, there can be a huge variability in terms of communication skills.

It is important to remember that some children with ASD will acquire language at the correct time, and this may appear to be typical. Previously children who had this profile (in addition to within average IQ) would have been diagnosed with 'Asperger's syndrome'. We know from Chapter One that this label is not used as a diagnostic anymore; however, some people with ASD still like to refer to themselves as 'Asperger's' or 'Aspie'.

We will now discuss some of the features of communication that you may see in a child with ASD. Just remember that all children will present differently in terms of their individual profiles of strengths and needs.

Communication skills

## Features of communication in ASD

What makes the communication skills of children with ASD different?

It isn't just that the communication skills of children with ASD are behind; they are following a different or 'disordered' pattern of development. Even when children with ASD have language, they can still communicate in a different or unusual way.

In Chapter One we discussed what you might see as some of the communicative features in a child with ASD. We turn now to illustrate this in more detail.

- **Difficulties in making requests** – This affects both children who don't have any language and also those that do. For example, a non-verbal child may show difficulties requesting – see Jack's case study as follows. Even when children have language, they may still struggle to 'ask' for things.

> **Case Study** Salma is four and a half. She has a diagnosis of ASD; she has been described as 'high functioning' with 'good language skills'. Although she has a detailed vocabulary, especially in relation to animals, which is one of her favourite topics, she finds it difficult to make requests. When she wants a drink, she will often ask an adult, 'Would you like a drink?' When stuck she will never ask for help. Recently her key worker noticed her doing a craft activity. When other children had the glue, she did not ask to have a turn and waited until it came near enough for her to reach over and take it.

- **Difficulties in understanding language** – Children with ASD may show a range of difficulties in understanding language. These may include the following:
  - Difficulties in following instructions
  - Spoken language that is better than understanding, for example, a child who talks in long sentences but doesn't appear to understand them
  - Difficulties in understanding non-literal language

- **Difficulties with joint attention** – Many early intervention programmes look to develop these skills in young children with ASD.

- **Lack of gestures** – If a child has a speech and language difficulty, he or she tries to send you a message using many means, for example, gestures and pointing. Children with ASD tend to use less-descriptive gestures, for example, using an action for drink as well as less conventional gestures, for example, shrugging, nodding, and shaking his or her head and waving as a greeting.

- **Difficulties with understanding and using non-verbal communication** – This may include facial expressions, tone, volume and rate of speech, body language, and touching.

- **Echolalia (repeated language)** – This may occur immediately when you ask a child 'Do you want a drink?' Instead of saying yes or no, they say 'Do you want a drink?' Echolalia can also occur later, for example, repeating a whole story or television programme. Often echolalia can mean that we overestimate the language abilities of a child. See activity sheet (C14) on top tips to reduce echolalia (repeated language).

- **Lack of social language** – Children with ASD may not engage in social chit-chat and conversation in a typical way. You probably won't notice them offering information about themselves unless it relates to a topic of their interests.

*Case Study:* Tom is three years old. He has a diagnosis of ASD; he is interested in other children and likes to run up to them. Tom will get close to their faces and shout, 'No pushing'. He then smiles and waits. He seems to want to engage with the other children but doesn't know how to do it. He doesn't have the appropriate social language to do so.

- **Stereotyped language** – This may occur when a child uses phrases and words that he or she has heard elsewhere. This can give his or her language a slightly unusual quality, for example, a child saying, 'I don't believe it'.

*Case Study:* Yafet is four years old. He has a diagnosis of ASD and has made a lot of progress with his language skills. He is now able to communicate in sentences. However, when adults listen closely to the language that Yafet is using, they realise that a lot of it is learnt from his favourite book, The Gruffalo. Yafet also echoes words that he has heard from favourite television programmes and also the routine at nursery, for example, 'Good job, Yafet'.

## What can we do to help?

We now turn to consider how we can help children with ASD develop their communication skills.

*TIP:* Communication is everywhere! You don't need to have a special time of day to carry out these activities, and many can be built into your everyday routines.

Remember, communication is much more than words. Many of the activities we now discuss are not focussing specifically on 'talking'. From our discussion of typical

# Communication Skills

development, you are aware that there are a lot of other skills that children need to develop to become effective communicators.

When you are working on joint attention and non-verbal communication, for example, you are helping to lay important foundation skills for a child. You can help parents understand this by explaining that we are working on 'communication fundamentals'. Often 'not talking' is one of the main things parents are worried about in their children. There is sometimes a tendency to focus on teaching a child using flash cards or focussing on descriptive words such as colours and numbers. Whilst these activities do have their place, it is important to develop all of a child's communication.

## Key components of communication – requesting

When I visit a child in an education environment, I always ask staff working with the child and the child's parents, 'How does he ask for things?' or 'How does he tell you which one he wants?' I am never surprised by the response; often staff working with a child may say, 'He doesn't really ask', or 'He is so independent. . . . He just gets everything himself'. Parents tend to respond, 'We know what he wants so he doesn't really need to ask'.

Imagine yourself in a foreign country – if you couldn't speak the language, one of the first things you would learn to communicate would be to tell others your basic needs. In the same way, children with ASD will be most motivated to communicate what they want. This has the benefit of reducing frustration and increasing confidence.

Requesting is key to developing communicative competence. Many interventions for children aim to teach children to make requests. Remember that a child can make requests both verbally and non-verbally.

Recognising that you can do a lot to help a child ask for things is important.

This can be extremely powerful for a child, as illustrated by Jack's case study.

**Case study: supporting Jack's requesting**

We talked about supporting Jack's understanding in Chapter Two. Let's recap and look at how staff working with Jack supported his ability to make requests.

### Background

Jack started nursery at age two and a half; at this time he was non-verbal with little response to any spoken language. When he started nursery he became upset whenever an adult attempted to direct him onto an activity or take him to change his nappy or wash hands and would only engage with cars lying down watching them at eye level. He didn't participate in the routines of the nursery and was self-directed. Staff working with him were keen to help him engage more so that he could access new and different learning opportunities.

Jack was unable to ask for anything and would communicate by screaming and pushing items away. He occasionally took an adult's hand to lead to the area where he wanted something and would reach towards a preferred item. Often Jack would climb to reach what he wanted and became frustrated when unable to communicate.

### Difficulty in requesting – what is the problem?

Jack has difficulties with 'asking'. He is beginning to understand that he can send a message to another person, for example, by taking his or her hand or reaching towards something. Most of the time he tries to get what he wants, and when he can't he becomes upset. The impact of this is significant; Jack can become distressed when unable to tell others what he wants. Jack's mother finds it difficult to take him places due to his frequent tantrums.

### What can we do to help?

Jack needs to learn how to make requests. To do this he needs adults working with him to help him.

### Change yourself, not the child

By changing the environment as described in Chapter Two and also how we communicate with young children with ASD, we can have a big impact.

### Actions

Staff got to know Jack and completed the Information-Gathering Tool (I-1) and Skills Profile (I-2). From this they were able to identify his profile of strengths and needs. Staff met with Jack's parents to discuss targets. Parents and staff agreed on the following targets (to support expressive skills and in particular requesting):

# Communication Skills

**Targets**

- For Jack to 'ask' for a favourite object when adults create chances for him to communicate
- For Jack to reach for a favourite object when offered a choice
- For Jack to 'give' an item to ask for help
- For Jack to vocalise for 'go' as part of ready, steady, go game

**Strategies used**

Staff working with Jack consistently used the following strategies:

- Offering choices of a preferred and non-preferred snack twice a day (C4)
- Offering choice
- Making chances for Jack to give items in play activities
- As described in Chapter Two, focussing on using consistent language – language for routines (E8), which meant that Jack was frequently hearing repeated words and phrases
- Helping Jack understand the concept of 'finished' (E4)
- Because this particular group of staff were quite musical, introducing a routine song for different activities including tidying up, snack time, shoes on off, as well as showing an object

**The results**

In three months Jack has shown improvements in his ability to ask for things. He does not yet communicate using words but is much less frustrated as he is clearly able to send a message in a number of ways.

- Jack is able to make a choice by reaching; he also makes a sound to indicate the item he wants.
- Jack consistently gives items to show that he wants them. For example, he will give an adult the bubbles when he wants an adult to blow them. Jack loves musical toys, but he can't start the wind-up toy on his own, so now knows to give it to an adult to play. He will make a sound for 'go'.

We will turn now to consider specific activities to support the communication skills in children with ASD in activity sheets (C1)–(C16).

# Communication skills

## Communication activity sheet 1. Developing joint and shared attention

**C:1**

**Without joint and shared attention, any two-way communication is going to be difficult for a child. We need to start with these skills to provide a foundation for communication skills to develop.**

*The Attention Autism programme is an extremely helpful approach in providing practical ideas to develop joint and shared attention and early communication skills. See www.ginadavies.co.uk for further information.*

### How to develop joint and shared attention

- Start off by observing the child you are working with. Pay attention to what he or she is interested in. Using a child's interests is the best starting place.

- Think about what stage of attention he or she is at on the Skills Profile. If a child is single channelled, he or she will need you to join in the activity.

- Join the child in the activity rather than trying to impose your activity.

- Tailor the activity to the child's interest.

### What skills are you looking for?

Working on joint attention can feel abstract; here are some of the skills that you are looking for a child to develop.

- A shared focus – looking at the same activity as you

- Sharing a focus – looking from the activity and back to you

- Responding when you look or point at something

- Pointing or looking at items to share interest

- Showing you things that are interesting to them (not asking you for them)

### Activities to develop joint attention

- Have an exciting bag of motivating objects that you take out and show the child. These may be light-up toys, bubbles, or whatever is motivating to the child. You are

# Communication Skills

looking for the child to join the activity for a short period. Resist the temptation to try and get them to show other skills such as requesting.

- Put items in unusual places, for example, a big sticker on the window, or a favourite toy on the shelf. Emphasise your pointing to direct their attention to activities.

- Make a shared focus fun and exciting, and use your facial expressions and props to engage the child.

- Use materials with motivating sensory properties, for example, pouring sand, water, shaking, shredded paper, and so on. Consider what an individual child likes and tailor your activities to these; see (P2) for sensory play ideas.

## Materials needed

- Dependent on individual child

# Communication skills

## Communication activity sheet 2. The power of pausing

**C:2**

**Pausing is a powerful way to support communication. This is especially important for children with limited communication skills. When children don't communicate much, there is a tendency to overcompensate and talk a lot for them. By stepping back and pausing, we offer valuable opportunities for skills to develop.**

*The strategies in this activity sheet are adapted from Sussman, F. (2012).* More Than Words®: A Parent's Guide to Building Interaction and Language Skills for Children With Autism Spectrum Disorder or Social Communication Difficulties. *Toronto, Ontario: The Hanen Centre, with permission from The Hanen Centre. For more information about the More Than Words® programme and trainings, visit hanen.org.*

## When we pause we give a child . . .

- Time to process
- A chance to communicate
- A cue to understand that it is his or her chance to communicate

Activity sheets (C4) to (C8) all incorporate pausing as part of the strategies used.

## When you pause during an activity . . .

- Get down to the child's level.
- Be engaged – use your facial expression and gestures to show a child that you are pausing expectantly for him or her to respond. Rather than waiting with a neutral face, communicate to the child that you are waiting excitingly for something to happen. Imagine being a young child, and it is Christmas tomorrow. Think about how your face may appear.
- Pause at a key point during the activity.
- Think about what you want the child to do; for example, are you looking for him or her to communicate with you that he or she wants more? Remember to respond to

## Communication Skills

all of a child's attempts to communicate; this may be looking, body movements, or sounds.

- Remember there is no pressure on the child to do anything. You are pausing to give him or her a chance to.

> **TIP** Practise your pausing face!

By putting in pauses to our communication, we also slow down what we are saying and become more conscious of how and why we are communicating and interacting with a child.

# Communication skills

## Communication activity sheet 3.
## Imitation 'copy me'!

**C:3**

Imitation is a powerful communication strategy to use, especially with children who have limited communication skills. Imitation is a key part of an approach called intensive interaction that is frequently used with children and adults with ASD. Think of when you hold a little baby. He or she makes a sound, and we naturally coo back. Imitation is a natural way of supporting communication. The great thing is that you can do it anywhere and don't need any resources at all. Sometimes you can feel a little self-conscious; however, the more you can commit and be at the child's level, the more powerful your imitation will be.

Through imitating a child's sounds and actions, we are helping him or her understand that his or her communication is powerful and has an impact on other people.

*For more information on intensive interaction, see www.intensiveinteraction.org.*

## Through imitating a child we can help a child to . . .

- Have a shared focus
- Take simple turns in an activity
- learn to imitate you (although this is not the goal)
- Engage with you in a non-pressured way

## How to imitate

- Start off by watching the child – what is he or she interested in?
- Join the child in the activity rather than trying to get him or her to do your activity.
- Be face to face.
- Follow his or her interests and what he or she is doing.
- Copy sounds and actions.
- Pause to see how the child responds.

## Communication Skills

- Keep the interaction going – make it fun.
- Remember there is no pressure for the child to 'do anything' in particular. You are providing an opportunity for shared focus and time to communicate.
- You may feel silly to start with, but it is worth making the effort.

### How to step it up

- Once you have established a shared focus, try adding in something new.

### Materials needed

- None

Communication Skills

## Communication activity sheet 4.
## Making chances to communicate – offering choices

C:4

**Offering choices is a useful way to help children make requests and 'ask for things'. By offering a choice we can help a child to show what he or she wants and reduce frustration. Choice making also provides an opportunity for modeling language and communicative behaviours such as reaching, pointing, and looking. By offering choices to children who have language, we are reducing the number of direct questions we ask and providing an opportunity to model new language.**

*The strategies outlined in activity sheets (C4)–(C6) are adapted from Sussman, F. (2012). More Than Words®: A Parent's Guide to Building Interaction and Language Skills for Children With Autism Spectrum Disorder or Social Communication Difficulties. Toronto, Ontario: The Hanen Centre, with permission from The Hanen Centre. For more information about the More Than Words® programme and trainings, visit hanen.org.*

## How to offer choices

- Start off by offering a choice between motivating and un-motivating items; that is, offer the child a choice between what he or she wants and something he or she is less interested in. This means that the child will communicate what he or she wants rather than reaching for both or losing interest.

- Clearly say what each option is; for example, say, 'Do you want ball or book?' whilst holding each item forward. This means that the child is hearing the single word whilst hearing the object.

- Your child may choose by looking, reaching, making a sound, or using the word to communicate which one he or she wants.

- As soon as the child indicates which item he or she wants, give it immediately, saying the name of the object he or she chose.

## When to offer choices

You can offer choices at any time of day.

In nursery this can be a good strategy to use consistently at certain times of the day, for example, snack time, song choosing during circle time, or before going out to the playground.

### How to step it up

- Choice making is a useful strategy to use even when children can tell you what they would like.

- You can offer choices including new and different concepts. This gives the opportunity to hear new words and also to practise saying them. For example, if you are working on size concepts, 'Would you like a *big* apple or a *little* apple?'

- Remember, as a child develops his or her language, you can use choices in relation to different words and actions see (C12); for example, if you are targeting a child's use of action words, try 'Shall we kick or throw the ball?'

### Materials needed

- No resources needed to offer verbal choices, just the objects you are choosing between

# Communication Skills

## Communication activity sheet 5.
## Making chances to communicate – giving

**C:5**

**Typically, young children will give an item as a way of getting an adult help or attention. Children with ASD do not typically do this. Creating chances for children with ASD to give is an easy way to facilitate requesting in the classroom. This is a great strategy as it is easy to implement and can be used effectively for children with little communication.**

### How to encourage children to give items

- Start off by paying attention as to whether the child already gives anything at all. You may notice that he or she gives a toy when he or she can't work it or when he or she is unable to open something – these are positive starts.

- Find out what his favourite interests are as he or she will be most motivated to communicate for these.

- A child with ASD is much more likely to give you an item that he or she needs help with as opposed to sharing an interest.

- With this in mind, use toys or items that the child needs help with or can't operate.

- Give the child a cue by offering your outstretched hand. To start off with, a child may throw or push the item towards you, but as he or she develops this skill, you will notice him or her giving, vocalising, and showing increased eye contact.

- If they don't give you the item, offer a hand-over-hand prompt. Remember to keep it fun at all times.

### *Example: bubbles – giving to ask more*

1. Blow a few bubbles to get the child's interest. Make it fun; pop them to get his or her interest.

2. Put the lid on the bubbles too tight so that the child will be unable to open them.

3. Place the bubbles nearby and pause.

4. Offer your outstretched hand as a cue. When the child gives you the bubbles, say 'Bubbles', and immediately blow them.

# Communication Skills

*Why would we say bubbles rather than thank you or more?* It is much better to teach the child the word for the object rather than a more abstract term, particularly for children with limited language.

## Example: in the box – giving to ask to open

1 Place a highly motivating toy or snack in clear Tupperware where the children can see it but can't access it.

2 Open the box, let them play for a short while and have a small snack, then place it back in the box.

3 Wait to see how they communicate they would like more. Offer your outstretched hand, and wait for them to give it to you.

## When to practise giving

Try this at any time of the day, although avoid times of tiredness or frustration.

## How to step it up

As a child becomes familiar with giving items, your goal may extend from giving you the item to giving and looking at you or giving and saying the word.

## Materials needed

- Clear plastic boxes
- Motivating toys and objects

# Communication activity sheet 6.
# Making chances to communicate – a bit at a time

**C:6**

**Naturally as parents and educators, we want to meet children's needs. For example, if we know that children like raisins, it makes sense to give them a bowl of raisins at snack time. We want them to be happy and enjoy the raisins.**

*But*, we can make many everyday activities into an opportunity for requesting by offering things a little at a time. Instead of giving everything all at once, give a few pieces, and wait to see how a child asks you for more. Depending on the level of communication, a child may reach, point, make a sound, or say a word to communicate with you that he or she wants more.

## This strategy works well in the following activities

With all these activities you could also use photographs to support understanding as outlined in (E2); for example, stick a photo of the snack on the Tupperware container or a photo of a puzzle piece on the bag containing the puzzle.

### *Snacks*

- Instead of leaving snacks out offer a few pieces at a time. Keep snacks in a Tupperware container. This also encourages giving (C5).

### *Puzzles*

- Use a plastic wallet with a zip to keep puzzles in. Offer a few pieces, and wait to see how the child 'asks' you for more.

### *Train tracks*

- Keep hold of a few pieces of train track, and wait to see how the child 'asks' you for more.

**Activity:** Think about what other activities in your environment lend themselves to offering a bit at a time.

### Communication skills

### How to step it up

Think about your expectations for the child. For a non-verbal child, it may be that you would like him or her to reach towards the piece. To step the activity up as he or she becomes familiar with it, you may have an expectation for him or her to reach and make a sound or reach and look at you. Similarly, for a child with words, you may expect him or her to say a word and look at you or say two words, and so on. Just remember that in increasing your expectations, it is important that a child is not feeling pressured or tested in any way.

### Materials needed

- Toys
- Plastic boxes and wallets
- Photographs where appropriate

# Communication Skills

## Communication activity sheet 7. Ready, steady, go games

C:7

**Playing ready, steady, go games can be a useful way to get a child to send you a message that he or she wants the game to start. The aim is for a child to send you a message to indicate 'go'. This may be by looking, making a sound, using body movements, or saying 'go'.**

## How to play a ready, steady, go game

- Think about an activity that the child may find motivating. Start with a game that he or she already enjoys.
- Start the game, for example, blowing a few bubbles or building a tower.
- Use facial expressions and tone to create interest and excitement.
- Say, 'Ready, steady . . . go'.
- Pause and wait expectantly to give the child a chance to request.
- Remember to wait expectantly and excitedly! To start off, you may need to wait for at least five to ten seconds.
- Respond to any attempt to communicate made by the child, for example, looking, reaching, or making a sound.

## You can incorporate ready, steady, go into lots of favourite games

**Bubbles:** Instead of blowing the bubbles continuously, blow a few bubbles. Wait and say, 'Ready, steady . . . go'! Wait for the child to show you how he or she wants you to blow the bubbles. He or she may look, reach, make a sound, or look. Repeat several times.

**On the swing:** Pull the swing back, and say, 'Ready, steady . . . go'! Wait for your child to show you how he or she wants you to release the swing. He or she may wriggle, vocalise, or try to say go.

**Knocking over a tower:** Slowly build a tower either together or with the child watching you in anticipation. Say, 'Ready, steady . . . go'! Repeat several times.

## Communication Skills

**Pull back cars and wind-up toys:** The advantage of these toys is that they can be hard to operate so that the child may give you them as well to start the game (C3).

*Activity* — Think of children you work with. What could you use as a ready, steady, go game with them?

## Materials needed

- Toys to use as part of the ready, steady, go game

# Communication skills

## Communication activity sheet 8. Stop/go games

C:8

The principles of a stop/go game are similar to ready, steady, go games (C7).

Stop/go games can be highly motivating for children and also provide an opportunity for them to be in control and use their voice. I have seen children with significant communication difficulties initiate go by moving their bodies and smiling. These are motivating activities that also provide a great opportunity for joint attention (C1).

## How to play a stop/go game

- Decide what you are going to stop go. This will depend on the child's motivation and interest.

- Start the game, for example, shaking the parachute, saying ready, steady, go'... pausing, and saying, 'Stop'. Hold your hands up in a gesture to show 'stop'.

- Say, 'Ready, steady ... go' and wait for the child to start the activity again (as outlined in C5).

- Use facial expressions and tone to create interest and excitement.

- Pause and wait expectantly to give the child a chance to request.

- Remember to wait expectantly and excitedly! To start off, you may need to wait for at least five to ten seconds.

- Respond to any attempt to communicate made by the child, for example, looking, reaching, and making a sound.

- Be consistent in your words and gestures that you use as part of the game. Repetition will help a child learn the steps of the game.

## Ideas for stop/go games

**Pouring:** Pouring can be highly visual and motivating for some children. Use a stop/go game when pouring water at the water table or sand at the sand tray. Get creative

## Communication Skills

and think about what else you can pour, for example, rice onto a tray or coloured water onto a tray.

**Shaking a parachute:** Parachutes are a great resource to use for lots of activities.

**Shaking a tinfoil blanket:** I use tinfoil blankets a lot as part of games, firstly because they are extremely cheap and durable and, secondly, they add a level of excitement and motivation for children who like sensory play. They make a great noise and visual display. Either sit the child you are working with on the blanket and shake/stop around him or her, or get him or her to hold the blanket and be involved in shaking.

## How to step it up

For children who are learning more language, add in concepts; for example, 'Shall we go fast/slow, high/low (shaking blanket)?' Be creative. Remember to keep language to the child's level.

## Materials needed

- Toys to use as part of the stop/go game

Communication skills

## Communication activity sheet 9. Making choices with a choosing board

C:9

(C4) outlines the importance of offering choices. Choice making is an easy strategy to incorporate into the environment to help children to make requests throughout the day. Often it is relatively easy to use the real objects when making a choice, for example, snack items or choosing different-coloured paper in a craft activity. Sometimes it can be harder to have all the items there to choose from. On these occasions it may be useful to use a choosing board.

## What is a choosing board?

A board made of a laminated card with a selection of attached photos, line drawings, or symbols. The choosing board is a visual representation of objects that a child may like to choose but can't communicate those choices (see Figure 3.1).

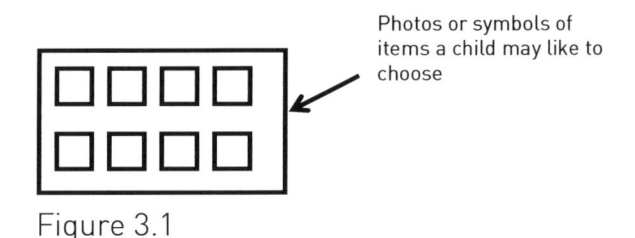

Photos or symbols of items a child may like to choose

Figure 3.1

## When to use

When to use a choosing board is likely to vary depending on the child and his or her individual interests. Certain activities (particularly those in which objects may not be available at the time) lend themselves to a choosing board, for example:

**Song choice:** Use a picture representation for songs at circle time so that a non-verbal child is able to make a choice when he or she is unable to respond verbally.

**Outside play:** An outside play choosing board could have photos of different equipment in the playground, for example, bike, ball, and scooter.

Before going outside, present the board and encourage a child to choose what he or she would like to play with.

**Snack:** A snack choosing board could have snack options on it.

**Musical instrument:** This version would include photos of different instruments.

**Communication Skills**

### How to use

- Offer the child the board – keep your language consistent; for example, 'I choose . . .' Or 'I like . . .' Try not to ask, 'What do you want?'

- Start off with two pictures on the board – to begin with, have a photo of an item that the child is not interested in so that you help him or her to make a clear choice.

- Once the child has made a choice, give him or her the item straightaway.

### Materials needed

- Photos or symbols
- Laminator
- Hook-and-loop fastener

## Communication activity sheet 10. Asking for help

**C:10**

**Being able to ask for help is an incredibly useful tool. Children may request help in a variety of ways, for example, by bringing you an item that he or she can't operate by giving it to you. Some children don't realise that they can send you a message to request help; this can then cause them to become frustrated. Asking for help is relevant for all children with ASD regardless of verbal level. As we discussed earlier in Chapter Three, 'asking' can be difficult for children with ASD. I have worked with non-verbal children who in frustration have just thrown items that they can't ask for help with and verbal children who instead of asking have sat and said to themselves, 'I can't do it'.**

**We can adapt the environment and create chances to enable children to successfully ask for help. This has the added benefit of meeting a need and reducing frustration.**

We need to create chances for a child to ask for help. This very much draws on the strategies outlined in (C2)–(C5). If we are able to set up these opportunities, we can 'teach' the child to 'ask' for help. Remember the way that a child asks you for help will depend on his or her verbal level. For example, a child with limited verbal communication may give you the item, whereas a child with more language may say, 'Help', or 'Help, please'.

### How to create chances to ask for help

- Select a motivating activity for the child; he or she won't be motivated to ask for help unless it is interesting or motivating.

- Make a chance for him or her to communicate, for example, by putting the lid on too tight or by using a jigsaw that is too hard to complete on his or her own.

- When they try to do it themselves, offer a cue; for example, extend outstretched hand and say, 'Help, please'.

- Pause and wait to see how the child asks you; this may be by giving you the item. Continue to model the useful phrase 'Help' or 'Help me, please', dependent on language level.

### Communication Skills

- Don't ask the child to repeat you or say, 'Say help me, please'. Don't ask questions such as 'Do you need help?' For some children who use repeated language, this will then become the phrase that they use.

## When to ask for help

Asking for help can be tailored to a range of activities. Easy ones within the early years environment include snack time or play activities.

## Materials needed

- Toys that are motivating but too hard for children to operate themselves

## Communication activity sheet 11. Using songs

C:11

In Chapter Two, we talked about how we can use songs to support understanding of routines. Music can be a powerful motivator, so we can use this across activities to support a wide range of communication skills for children who are verbal and non-verbal. Songs and rhymes are great ways to develop communication skills in children with ASD and all SLCN. Rather than singing the songs, we can use some of the following key strategies to help a child communicate.

## How to use songs to support communication

- **Start the song the same way** – Use a consistent gesture, word, or action. You may add a visual cue such as an object or symbol; for example, say, 'Row, row', show the boat, and put your hands outstretched.

- **Be face to face** – Being at a child's level is important to support communication. This might mean sitting or lying on the floor. It also means that you can see all of the child's attempts to communicate with you; you are then ideally placed to respond straightaway.

- **Respond to and interpret all of a child's attempts to communicate** – This may be eye contact, a wiggle, a smile, or a sound. When you respond immediately and continue the song, this helps a child learn about sending messages to make things happen.

- **Pause during key points** – In (C2) we talked about how pausing and waiting is an important strategy as it gives a child the opportunity to ask for more. A child may ask for more by looking at you, reaching for your hands, or vocalizing. Pause during exciting parts of the song, for example, in 'Row, Row, Row Your Boat' just before the scream. Pause and wait to see if a child fills in the sound or word.

- **Incorporate movement and props to create anticipation** – During 'Zoom Zoom' after five, four, three, two, one, lift your child up, pause, and create anticipation.

- **Think about how the child you are working with is going to ask you for more and offer cues to help this** – In 'Round and Round the Garden Like a Teddy Bear', pause

# Communication Skills

and offer your hand. Your child may reach for your hand to communicate he or she wants more. As he or she becomes used to the routine, he or she may reach for your hand and make a sound or use a word.

**Activity** — Think of a child and a song that he or she likes, use the following checklist to break the song down to support communication:

- How will you start the song, for example, with a sound, word, and/or gesture?
- How will you create chances to communicate; for example, pause at an exciting point?
- How will you finish the song?

## How to step it up

For children who regularly join in songs, you could add choices with different concepts; for example, 'Shall we sing loud or quiet/fast or slow?'

## Materials needed

- Objects or pictures to represent songs (optional)

# Communication skills

## Communication activity sheet 12. Adding language

**C:12**

Even when children aren't talking, they are often listening and learning language. Being able to add language to your activities and interaction is a helpful way to support understanding and expression. SLTs often call this 'modeling language'. We can think about the types of words we use and also what functions we are using them for.

## Cut the questions

- As adults we ask a lot of questions, even to children who can't necessarily respond. Instead of asking questions, you can make comments and model language to support a child's communication.

**Activity** Time yourself in an interaction with a child for ten minutes, and consciously count the number of questions you ask. In most cases you will be surprised it's a lot more than you think!

## Add helpful words

- Think about words that are useful for the child, for example, rather than using words without a specific meaning, such as 'that one' and 'there'. Use the specific word.

- Don't add labels – add action words (C13).

- Add social language, for example, 'Let's play, my turn' (S5).

**TIP** 'Say it as if he/she could' is a useful rule when modeling language.

## Communicate at the child's level

- Be at a child's physical level when you are talking to him or her.

- Model language at the right level; for example, if a child is using no words and we talk in long sentences, it is too much for them to take on. For example, for a child with limited language, saying, 'Look over there. It's a red bus. You like buses', doesn't help the child see the bus and learn the word 'bus'. Instead be at the child's

## Communication Skills

level, point to the bus, say, 'bus', and repeat several times. If the child then makes an attempt to say bus, you then add a word: 'red bus'.

Think about how you can change a question into a comment and add useful language (see Figure 3.2). For example, Jack is playing with the train.

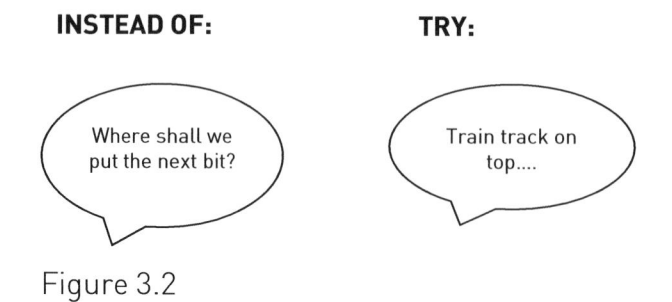

**INSTEAD OF:**       **TRY:**

*Where shall we put the next bit?*      *Train track on top....*

Figure 3.2

# Communication Skills

## Communication activity sheet 13. Using action words

**C:13**

**Learning action words are an important part of language development. They are key to linking words together and making longer sentences. If a child knows lots of nouns, for example, dog, water, and ball, it is difficult to link words to make a sentence; for example, dogs *drink* water. Action words are key building blocks in language. Often children with ASD have large labeling vocabularies but struggle with using everyday action words. Developing action words is an important area to focus on.**

## Ideas and activities to try

- The great thing about action words is that they occur in everyday activities when you are 'doing things'.

- Make a verb book; take photos of the child you work with and other children doing different activities; for example, 'Jack is sleeping' or 'Grace is eating'. These pictures will be fun and motivating to make comments on. Children are often more motivated by pictures of themselves.

- Use practical activities during which you make and do things, for example, cooking (mix and pour) or snack time (cut fruit, drink, and eat).

- When you are looking at pictures in books, instead of just labeling the pictures, talk about what the people are doing.

- Try not to test your child, for example, asking, 'What are they doing?' Instead make comments at the time they are happening; for example, 'Mummy is eating and Jack is eating'.

- Add to and expand what the child is saying with an action word; for example, when he or she comments, 'Look, dog', you say, 'Yes, the dog is running'.

- Choose several action words to focus on each week, and comment on these in everyday activities. Remember that when learning new words, children need lots of repetition across different activities and contexts.

## Communication Skills

- Start off with everyday, common verbs, for example, eat, drink, sleep, and jump, before moving onto more abstract verbs such as pull, pour, hop, and so on.
- Use natural gestures to reinforce understanding, and give a visual cue.
- Once you feel the child understands the verbs, you can give choices in activities to help him or her use the words; for example, when playing with the ball, ask, 'Shall Mummy kick the ball or throw the ball?'

### Materials needed

- Photographs (only for verb book)

## Communication activity sheet 14. Reducing repeated language

**C:14**

**As we discussed earlier in this chapter, children with ASD will often show echolalia as part of their communication. Echolalia is where children repeat what has been said. This may occur immediately, for example, when you say 'What is your name', the child repeats what you have said. Some children may hear something that they echo later. Sometimes children will echo words that they have heard from a favourite programme, and at other times their echoing may be trying to tell you something; for example, when a child says 'Would you like a drink', when they want a drink.**

**Sometimes the use of echolalia means that we overestimate a child's language abilities; children can use phrases that they don't fully understand. Echolalia can be helpful at times to help children learn new phrases and words; just remember, some children echo without understanding the meaning of what they are saying.**

*The strategies in this activity sheet are adapted from Sussman, F. (2012).* More Than Words®: A Parent's Guide to Building Interaction and Language Skills for Children With Autism Spectrum Disorder or Social Communication Difficulties. *Toronto, Ontario: The Hanen Centre, with permission from The Hanen Centre. For more information about the More Than Words® programme and trainings, visit hanen.org.*

There are lots of ways that we can help children reduce echolalia. This needs you to be a detective and try to understand what a child is trying to communicate and replace it with a more appropriate phrase or action.

By adding helpful language at a child's level (C12) and reducing the number of questions that we ask, we are already providing the appropriate language for a child to pick up on.

## Tips to reduce repeated language

- **Watch carefully to see what a child is communicating** – Once you understand what he or she is trying to tell you, it is much easier to offer an appropriate language model. For example, if he says 'Do you want a biscuit', watch what other

## Communication Skills

communication he or she is using, such as leading you towards the biscuits or reaching for a biscuit. Once you realise that he or she actually wants a biscuit, you can respond.

- **Respond to what the child is trying to tell you** – They are sending you a message (even though the words may be incorrect), and it is important that we respond to what they are trying to tell us.

- **Say it as if he or she could** – This involves you talking from the child's point of view; for example, 'I want a biscuit'. Try to avoid saying his or her name as this will sound unusual if the child then repeats this him- or herself.

# Communication skills

## Communication activity sheet 15. Let's create

**C:15**

I have always found using creative everyday activities where you 'make' something a motivating way to work on language and communication skills in children with ASD. Working on an activity with a sequence gives lots of opportunities to add language (C12) and work on action words (C13), as well as provide opportunities for requesting (C4–C8) with an added bonus of providing a shared and joint focus of attention (C1).

*For further creative and practical activities to support early communication skills I would recommend the Attention Autism programme.*

## Activity ideas

- Make a sandwich.
- Make play dough – once you have made your play dough, add glitter to make it sparkly.
- Prepare a snack – make a fruit salad.
- Tailor activity to the child's interests; for example, if he or she enjoys sensory exploratory play, try some of the ideas in (P2).

## Top tips

- Talk about what is happening in the order that it is happening, for example, first, then, next.
- Make it visual; you can also take photos of the activity and use for teaching new language and sequences (C12). The photos also are a great context for discussion and sharing what a child has been done as part of a 'chat book'.
- Use language at the correct level. The great thing about creative activities is that they are motivating; it is about adding the right level of language. You may use the same activity, for example, making play dough with two different children, but your

## Communication Skills

expectation of what each child will do will be different. This goes back to the key philosophy of *'change yourself and not the child'*.

*Activity* — Think about making play dough with Jack and Lucille, who we met in Chapter One. You can use the same activity with different aims and expectations for each child. Consider the following key points to help you plan the activity:

- What is the activity?
- What do I need?
- What do I want 'the child to do'?
- What strategies can I use to support this?
- How can I start the activity?
- How can I finish the activity?

## Materials needed

- Planning sheet in Appendix Three

## Communication activity sheet 16. Using an about-me book

**C:16**

**Many children with ASD find it difficult to share information about themselves even if they have the language skills. Providing a context can be a great way to make this easier for them. This can be by using an about-me book. This can help a child 'offer' information about themselves, which is a good way to start conversations. For a child who doesn't have language, he or she may like looking at the pictures with you, which can provide a shared focus.**

## What is an about-me book?

An about-me book (or communication passport, as they are often known) provides information and pictures about a child, his or her family, favourite toys, and activities so that they have a context to talk about these things.

## Using an about-me book

For more verbal children, you could extend the book into a sharing news book in which parents stick or draw pictures of what they have done during the weekend and the same from the nursery day. All children find it difficult to answer that 'What did you do today?' question; we know that children with ASD have strengths in their visual skills, so providing this context gives them more of a chance to succeed in sharing information about themselves (which is also quite difficult).

## How to make an about-me book

You can use an A5 folder or spiral-bound laminated sheets. Use pictures and symbols. It can be helpful when making the book to involve a child's parents/carers so that they can have a similar one at home.

The following pages are useful:

- Me and my family
- My favourite things
- Places I like to go
- I like to talk about . . .
- Over the weekend I did . . .

## Materials needed

- Resources to make about-me book

## Communication Skills

> **Chapter Three summary**
>
> - Communication is a core difficulty for children with ASD.
>
> - Each child with ASD that you meet will communicate in a different way, which means that their strengths and needs will be different. We need to tailor our understanding and approach to the individual child.
>
> - Sometimes the communication needs of children with ASD mean that they can be perceived as 'rude' or 'disinterested'.
>
> - Often when children with ASD can't communicate, this is expressed as behaviour.
>
> - Even when children can talk, they can present with communication difficulties.
>
> - Even for children with language, making requests can be difficult for children with ASD.

## References

Cooper, J., Moodley, M. and Reynell, J. (1978). *Helping Language Development: A Developmental Programme for Children with Early Learning Handicaps.* London: Edward Arnold.

# Chapter Four
# SOCIAL INTERACTION

**Chapter Four provides the following:**

- A recap of what social interaction difficulties may look like in children with ASD
- Practical case studies to guide your thinking
- Tips on how to support children to achieve success in the social environment
- Activity sheets:

    **(S1) – A shared social experience**

    **(S2) – A shared social focus**

    **(S3) – Making a chance to interact**

    **(S4) – Making interaction predictable by adding structure**

    **(S5) – Adding social language**

    **(S6) – Taking turns**

    **(S7) – Taking turns – making it visual**

    **(S8) – Using a turn-taking board**

    **(S9) – Let's chat – top tips for conversations**

    **(S10) – Understanding others; foundations of theory of mind**

## Social interaction: a core difficulty of ASD

From the theory you have read and case studies that you have worked through so far, you know that social interaction is a core difficulty for children with ASD. Like many features of ASD, the level of difficulty experienced by the individual child may vary, and this may change over time. We know that every

# Social interaction

child with ASD is different, so it makes sense that their profile of social interaction skills will also be unique to them. I have worked with an extremely wide range of children with ASD, from those who are sociable and interested in interaction but don't manage to get it quite right in terms of the right thing to say or understanding body language and tone of voice, to those who have no real awareness of other people. Regardless of the child's level, as educators it is so important to feel like you have the skills to support children in this area.

It is important to acknowledge that at times, working with children who struggle with social interaction can be challenging and often can leave practitioners feeling at a loss of where to start and what to do when their attempts to interact are met with little response.

All too often I have visited nurseries and asked who or what a child likes to play with to be met with a response, 'He's really happy on his own. He likes to do his own thing'. Whilst this may appear to be the case, we have a key role in making social interaction motivating and fun for children with ASD to engage in.

Being able to help children make connections and have a social focus is of key importance and can make a huge impact to those children and their families. I am often astounded at the small tweaks we need to make to our interaction to have a huge impact on a child. In my work with parents, I often have them doing all sorts of silly things that their child finds motivating. I will always remember working with a father who admittedly found it extremely hard to get a response from his child with ASD. His child knew colours and numbers and loved matching games but found it hard to engage in reciprocal interaction. Within a few weeks the father was crawling around the floor like a horse, playing chasing games and a game they had invented jumping on a cushion; his child was showing more eye contact and shared enjoyment, laughing, and requesting the interaction to continue. It was such a pleasure to observe and facilitate.

The social challenges and how these will unfold over time can be difficult to understand, particularly when children are young. Often parents ask about what the future holds for their children.

We know that with the right support, children with ASD are able to make progress in all areas, including social interaction. However, there may be times where difficulties

## Social interaction

become more significant, for example, transfer to secondary school or starting in a new setting. There may be other times when these areas of need are well managed.

This chapter looks in more detail at social interaction and provides practical ideas and strategies to support this. As mentioned in previous chapters, the areas that have been covered are closely related; for example, communication and interaction go hand in hand.

Remember that social communication and interaction difficulties are a core difficulty of ASD. Children's difficulties are not because they are being rude or naughty. Often when children with ASD communicate and behave in a different way from other children, this can lead to them being misunderstood. We look in more detail at this in Chapter Six when we focus on understanding behaviour. However, it is important to be aware that often we can misinterpret children with ASD. In addition to this there are a number of stereotypes and myths which persist around social interaction in ASD.

## Myths around social interaction

There are a lot of misconceptions around ASD; often these are routed in stereotypical views of ASD. Just because children with ASD have social interaction difficulties doesn't mean they don't want to be social.

- Children with ASD don't want friends – MYTH. Many children with ASD that I work with do want friends and form close bonds with other children. Structure and predictability can help interactions be easier and more successful for children.

- Children with ASD are not affectionate – MYTH.

- Children with ASD are not interested in other people – MYTH.

*Activity:* Go back to the "Milestones That Matter Most" from the FIRST WORDS PROJECT© in Chapter Three on pages 83–84. Think about how social interaction develops typically and how this is different for a child with ASD.

The following case studies illustrate some of the challenges with social interaction that children with a diagnosis of ASD face. It's worth thinking in detail about the social interaction profile of children in your setting who have diagnoses of ASD. This includes both areas of strength and areas of need.

Imagine how hard it must be for the child living in a world that is so social.

# Social interaction

> **Case Study**

**Lack of social response and reciprocity:** Lana is three years old; she has a diagnosis of ASD. She is non-verbal and has limited expressive communication. She has been at nursery for one year and has settled in well to the routine. She has a good relationship with her key worker and enjoys chasing games and songs which she will now initiate. She loves messy play activities, and staff are expanding her range of play using her interests. When Lana is excited she flaps her hands and vocalises.

A theatre group are coming to nursery and have a planned a group activity during with the children need to make a mask. When they arrive Lana is unable to sit and take part and walks away from the group. Later on she is excited by adult singing and waving scarves and joins in, running around and vocalising. The adult running the group has limited understanding of ASD and thinks Lana is badly behaved and rude.

> **TIP**

We all have a duty to spread awareness of ASD. When unfamiliar people are visiting your setting, let them know that you have a child with ASD. You could signpost them to the National Autistic Society website and, with parental consent, share a profile on the child. For an example of a profile, see Appendix Three.

> **Case Study**

**Difficulties with conversations:** Seren is four and a half; he has a detailed and rich knowledge and vocabulary relating to transport and planets. He talks at length about these topics and has limited understanding of having a conversation.

On a recent trip to a farm with a nursery, Seren talks at length with a parent volunteer about the machinery on the farm. He is unable to answer her questions and doesn't listen to what she says. The volunteer knows that he is different from the other children but finds it hard to find a way to engage with him.

> **Case Study**

**Style of communication:** Freddie is four years old. He has recently received a diagnosis of ASD. The paediatrician has mentioned that he has 'high-functioning ASD'. Freddie is verbal. He is able to engage in some conversations. Freddie has a flat tone of voice and speaks in a monotone. His face rarely changes even when he is excited or sad.

He recently went to a birthday party of a friend – one of the parents asked Freddie's mum if he wasn't having a nice time as 'he didn't look very happy'.

# Social interaction

**Case Study** — **Difficulties with non-verbal communication:** Ahmed is three and a half years old. He has a diagnosis of ASD. He receives OT support as he has sensory difficulties. Ahmed loves to hug people and will hold children at nursery tightly.

He recently tried to hug a stranger on the bus, which caused his mum concern.

**Case Study** — **Difficulties initiating in a typical way:** Rosa is four; she doesn't have a diagnosis of ASD but has been referred for assessment. Her difficulties are subtle as she appears on the surface to join in; however, staff have increasingly noticed that often she will mimic what the other girls say. She has one particular friend, and if this child is not present, Rosa can appear a little lost. Rosa clearly wants to engage but at times seems unsure what to do. She watches the other children closely and will sometimes try and start an interaction; sometimes this is in a slightly unusual way, for example, stroking their hair.

## Why is social interaction so challenging?

- Poor theory of mind
- Difficulties with understanding
- Sensory difficulties
- Unpredictable social interactions
- Core difficulties of social communication and interaction difficulties

All of these factors mean that being social (which most of us just take for granted) is difficult.

But there is lots that we can do to help.

## Supporting social interaction in the early years

In the early years there is much that can be done to give young children with ASD:

- Social opportunities
- Positive social experiences
- Opportunities for shared enjoyment with peers

# Social interaction

Even though 'social interaction' is a separate chapter, it is very much linked to the previous chapters. The strategies outlined in Chapter Two and Chapter Three also support interaction. It makes sense that if you are more relaxed in your environment and able to communicate to a greater degree, you are more able to be sociable.

In Chapter Three we talked about joint and shared attention and how we could establish these (C1) using motivating activities and also imitation (C3). Making a connection with a child is of key importance to developing early communication and interaction skills.

## Tips for making a connection

- Consider what the children are interested in and join them in their activity rather than imposing your own.
- Imitate (C3).
- Be playful and engage in fun, motivating games.
- Don't be self-conscious; the children you are working with will appreciate you getting down to their level and putting in the effort to connect with them.
- Get down to a child's level. This sounds like such a simple tip, but it makes all the difference. You may need to lie down on your front – whatever you need to ensure you are face to face. This is particularly relevant during books and songs; often we sit children on our knees facing outwards. Instead sit on the floor with your legs out and have the child sit facing you.

## Top tips for social interaction

- Say what you mean, and mean what you say – much of social interaction is reliant on non-verbal communication, which can be confusing for children with ASD. Where other children may pick up on more subtle social cues such as changes in an adults' facial expressions or tone of voice, a child with ASD may find this hard.
- Give clear language to accompany your facial expressions; this will help children make the social connection. Emotions can be abstract for children with ASD to process. If you can act as a guide and provide extra information about what is happening at the time it is happening, this can be helpful; for example, 'Salma, you

look really happy. I can see you are smiling. I think it is because you like playing with the dolls'.

- All of the communication strategies outlined in Chapter Three are extremely relevant for supporting social interaction. Naturally most of the activities that you do are targeting both areas; for example, during pauses you may find that as well as using a word to request, a child looks at you and smiles to share enjoyment.

- Be predictable in your interactions; to start off play games the same way. This gives children with ASD time to figure out what they are expected to do. Once the game is established you can introduce new elements or start to teach flexibility as part of the routine.

- Be realistic and give time to practise skills; for example, practise taking turns or a new game with an adult before expecting a child to do it in a small group with other children.

- Pausing is a powerful tool. Pause as part of interactions, and wait expectantly to give a child a cue to continue the game.

## What not to do

- One common 'don't do' that sometimes happens is when adults demand children with ASD to look at them. We know that eye contact can be challenging for some children. We want communication and interaction to be spontaneously joyful rather than being demanding of a child.

- Don't try to impose your agenda on a child and make him or her conform to what everyone else is doing. We need to change ourselves and not the child. Through changing ourselves, using positive strategies, and adapting our environment, we can have a positive impact on social communication and interaction skills.

- Try to avoid language around emotions; for example, 'It will make me very happy if you sit still'; most children with ASD in the early years will struggle to understand this, and also they won't be motivated by 'making an adult happy'.

- Don't leave children to focus on their own self-chosen activities, however happy they may be doing them.

- Don't take offence if a child doesn't respond to you in a typical way.

Social interaction

## Social interaction activity sheet 1. A shared social experience

S:1

**The very nature of a diagnosis of ASD means that social interaction can be challenging for children with ASD. However, just because interaction is difficult doesn't mean that children with ASD don't want to be social or can't enjoy social interaction. One of the major benefits of being around other children is the opportunity to engage in reciprocal interactions. As early years educators you are in an ideal position to facilitate positive social experiences for a child with ASD.**

**Some children may have had limited opportunities with other children, and those that they may have had (in the park or at toddler groups) may not have involved a shared and joint focus.**

### Involve children with ASD

This may sound silly; however, often I have visited children in an early years setting to consistently see them playing with their own activity in the same corner of the nursery. Having an expectation that a child with ASD will join in even for a short period is important. I have often been met with 'he can't do circle time', so the child is seldom included. Remember, 'change yourself, not the child'. Consider how you can adapt your circle time activity so that it is motivating for the child with ASD. One setting I visited did exactly this and decided to incorporate a parachute game at the end of every circle time.

### Involve other children

I was lucky to work in a wonderful ASD resource base attached to a mainstream school. The teacher included the mainstream children as helpers and partners for the children with ASD at every opportunity even to the point of teaching the children how to imitate. This worked well, and the non-verbal children with ASD responded far better to other children than an adult. Typical children love having a role; being a helper or showing another child can be highly motivating.

When a child with ASD has a shared social experience you may notice the following:

- Joining in the activity alongside other children
- Eye contact

- Smiling
- Shared enjoyment
- Joint and shared attention (C1)

Remember, the aim is to provide an opportunity and activity where these can happen.

## Activity ideas for a shared social experience

- Tailoring to the individual child and their preferences
- Music and dancing
- Parachute games

## Materials needed

- Tailored activities to the child's interests

Social interaction

## Social interaction activity sheet 2. A shared social focus

**S:2**

**Remember, social interaction starts with a shared social experience. I often emphasise the importance in having a child look at you, smile at you, and laugh in response to you. These are all important skills as part of social interaction. Sometimes we can get bogged down in trying to develop skills that are too hard. So often I visit children where there is an emphasis on taking turns and sharing; some children aren't ready for this, and there are important skills to focus on before this.**

To develop interaction you need to have a shared social focus. This overlaps with developing joint attention as outlined in (C1).

A shared social focus may involve the following:

- Focussing on the same activity, song, or interactive sequence
- Smiling
- Laughing
- Shared attention and enjoyment

Once you have a shared social focus you can do the following:

- Give meaning to a child's actions
- Engage in two-way, reciprocal interaction

In the Attention Autism programme, Gina Davies frequently talks about being 'the most exciting thing in the room'; this is of key importance to developing a shared social focus.

Throughout this manual we have emphasised the philosophy of 'change yourself, not the child' – you can adapt what you are doing in motivating interactions to give a child with ASD a chance to engage.

To start off with, a child may not come and ask you to play or interact. You can use strategies to get the child's interest and create a shared social focus:

- Get to the child's level.
- Imitate a child's actions, sounds, and movements (C3).

# Social interaction

- Be playful.
- Use their interests and preferences, for example, tickling or bouncing on your knee.
- Use pausing (C2).
- Slow down – this can be one of the most powerful strategies. Typically interaction happens so quickly and naturally. If we can slow down, we can help children with ASD join in, pick up on the cues that they need to learn to take a turn, and ultimately start the game with us.
- Repeat, repeat, repeat; a child with ASD will benefit from the activity happening many times so they become familiar with what is expected of them.

## Materials needed

- It can be useful to go back to the Skills Profile to consider the child's current levels.

Social interaction

## Social interaction activity sheet 3. Making a chance to interact

S:3

Once we have created a shared social focus, we can use strategies as part of motivating games and interactions to encourage a child to join in, request more, and start the game. As we mentioned at the beginning of Chapter Four, many strategies and activities that you have learnt in Chapter Three on communication are relevant to interaction. Rather than applying them to requesting objects, toys, or snacks, they can be applied to interaction. Recap activity sheets (C2), (C5), and (C7). We will look now at how we can apply the strategies of pausing, giving, and using a ready, steady, go game as part of an activity.

*The strategies in this activity sheet are adapted from Sussman, F. (2012).* More Than Words®: A Parent's Guide to Building Interaction and Language Skills for Children With Autism Spectrum Disorder or Social Communication Difficulties. *Toronto, Ontario: The Hanen Centre, with permission from The Hanen Centre. For more information about the More Than Words® programme and trainings, visit hanen.org.*

To make a chance for a child to interact we need to do the following:

- Slow the interaction down, and use the appropriate language level.
- Start the game the same way.
- Use consistent words, gestures, and props.
- Incorporate pauses.
- Finish the game the same way.

## Peekaboo

- **Start the game the same way** – Show the scarf, and put it on your head.
- **Use consistent words, gestures, and props** – Sing, 'Where is (your name)?'
- **Incorporate pauses** – Pause (the child may pull down the scarf), then you say, 'Boo'.
- **Finish the game the same way** – Say, 'five, four, three, two, one, hiding has finished' and put the scarf away.

As the children become familiar with the game, they may request more of the activity by giving (C5), for example, giving you the scarf to put on your head. When we pause (C2), we give them a chance to do this.

## Ready, steady, go

We talked about ready, steady, go games in (C7). This strategy lends itself nicely to tickling games or chasing games (and many more). Use your knowledge of a child to think about how you can incorporate this strategy.

- Start the game; for example, say 'Tickle', show a gesture, and then tickle toes.
- Use facial expressions and tone to create interest and excitement.
- Say, 'Ready, steady', wait with your hands poised to tickle, and the say, 'Go'.
- Pause and wait expectantly to see what happens.
- Children may say 'Go' or grab your hands or look at you to show that they want the tickling to continue.
- Remember to wait expectantly and excitedly. To start off, you may need to wait for at least five to ten seconds.
- Respond to any attempt to communicate made by the child, for example, looking, reaching, or making a sound.

## Materials needed

- See Appendix Five for an interaction planner.

Social interaction

## Social interaction activity sheet 4. Making interaction predictable by adding structure

**S:4**

**Social interactions can be unpredictable, which means that children with ASD can find it difficult to know what the expectations are, when they are supposed to take a turn, how to behave, and so on. By focussing on practical social games and routines, we can bring predictability to interactions to support children with their ability to take part consistently. We have discussed how important structure is to children with ASD. By bringing structure to interactions, we can support children with ASD to join in.**

### Add structure – communication strategies

- Use consistency as outlined in Appendix Four. Try applying this to the following games and activities:
- Peekaboo (as discussed)
- Chase me or 'I am going to get you . . .'
- Songs

### Add structure – environment

You can structure the environment to support interactions.

- Try playground games such as 'What's the Time, Mr Wolf' or 'throw the bean bag in the hoop'. Break the game down into component parts – you could break the game down and present this as outlined in (E12), or this could be drawn out on a whiteboard. Think about the physical structure (E10) and how you set up the game, for example, taping a line for the children to stand on. Have a spot to stand on if you are the wolf.

- Think about whether there are particular areas or times of day that lend themselves better to social interaction. This may vary per child.

### Add structure – visuals

- You can use visuals to support interaction, for example, a turn-taking board (S8).
- Use photographs to support understanding. Most education settings use photos to document a child's progress. You can add photos to their about-me books, or use

them as a tool to teach action words or even to reinforce positive behaviour and as a context for conversation. I worked with an able, verbal boy with ASD where the education setting used photographs nicely as part of small-group activities.

When working on any social interaction activity, remember that it has to be fun and motivating and to go at the child's pace.

## Materials needed

Go back to the Skills Profile to think about an individual child's strengths and needs so that you can tailor activities.

Social interaction

## Social interaction activity sheet 5. Adding social language

**S:5**

**In (C12) we talked about adding language. As well as adding descriptive language and action words to enrich a child's language, we can also add social language. Modeling the right language to a child during interaction is a positive way to develop social phrases. Many children who I have worked with have had goals around greetings; although saying hello and good-bye can be important, it isn't always the most useful phrase for a child to have. That doesn't mean not to encourage it; just be sure to include useful social language as well.**

*'He wants to play, he just doesn't know how'.*

This is a common theme I hear when visiting children with ASD in early years education. Often children with ASD are watching or attempting to join in but not in quite the right way. We can add social language to provide a model for children trying to engage.

As mentioned in (C12), the following strategies are useful:

- Say it as if the child could.
- In Chapter Six we talk about being a detective around a child's behaviour. There may be times when you need to do this to support interaction.
- Resist the temptation to ask the child to repeat you. Instead, model the phrase for them.

Useful social phrases to help children join in:

- My turn
- Let's play
- Let's go
- Chase me
- I'm going to get you

For children who have more language (are able to engage in a short conversation), model social language that helps them keep the conversation going:

- Commenting – I like it
- Questioning – What did you do over the weekend? Do you want to play with me?

# Social interaction

## When to use social phrases

- Model social phrases at the time when children need them, for example, when they are watching other children.

- Use them as a replacement; for example, if a child tries to grab a toy, gently say, 'My turn, please'.

- For children with more language, set up structured times to chat. This may be around a particular topic, for example, a favourite activity. I am interested that often, verbal children with ASD can do well with show-and-tell type activities. In many ways this makes sense, as there is a clear, predictable structure.

## Materials needed

- None

Social interaction

## Social interaction activity sheet 6. Taking turns

S:6

**Turn taking is often an area of focus for children with ASD. Turn taking can be difficult for all children, regardless of SLCN or SEND. Often we try to get children to take turns in activities that are too difficult for them, for example, a game with another child or handing over a toy. Taking turns and sharing actually involves numerous, quite complex thought processes which can be quite difficult for children with ASD. Being able to take turns in a specific game involves children being able to wait. Recap (E6) as this may be a useful cue to include when you are encouraging children to take turns. Turn taking starts a long way before sharing – you can take turns with children of all communication levels. Remember to adapt the activity to their interests and communication style.**

## Top tips for taking turns

- Vocal turn taking with an adult can be a great place to start and relates to (C2). When a child makes a sound, copy him or her. This non-pressured play activity is an easy way to take turns.

- Practicing with an adult first is important; although ultimately the goal is for a child to be able to take turns with another child, we can't guarantee that another child will respond how we want them to. So that the child with ASD has lots of positive opportunities, it can be useful to first engage with an adult.

- Use consistent language, for example, 'My turn'. You may introduce waiting as well as other visual supports such as a first/then board as a child becomes more familiar with the concept of taking turns. Use a gesture to indicate whose turn it is.

- Use quick games to start with. If a turn is taking too long and the child needs to wait too long, you can lose the focus of turn taking, and it becomes more about waiting. Quick turns allow a child to become involved quickly.

- Use a child's interests and motivations to keep it fun.

- Use predictable activities in which the turns are fairly consistent.

- Once a child is familiar with a turn-taking game, bring in other children.

- If you are using a prop or game as part of the interaction, make sure that it isn't too motivating for the child to just want to take the object and focus on it themselves.

## Social interaction

### Games for quick turn taking

- Roll a ball
- Bubbles for . . .
- Hiding (peekaboo with a scarf) – this also provides an opportunity for giving and for the child to initiate the game
- Cause-and-effect pop-up type toys
- Bricks for making a tower where you each take a turn

### Materials needed

- None for vocal turn taking and imitation
- Games for quick turn taking

Social interaction

## Social interaction activity sheet 7. Taking turns – making it visual

**S:7**

We know that taking turns is complicated for children with ASD. Turn taking involves complex social processes and understanding which can be challenging for children with ASD, especially those with no theory of mind. Remember the 'change yourself, not the child' philosophy. If we can change how we present turn-taking activities and our expectations of the child, we can enable children with ASD to achieve success in these activities. Adding visual supports and clear structure can make the game more predictable, reduce anxiety, and enable the child to engage.

### By adding structure to turn taking, we can help children understand

- Whose turn is it?
- How long is the turn going to be?

### What structure can we add?

- Wait card
- Turn-taking board (S8)
- Use of sand timers/countdown timers
- Use of a script or social story

*Activity* Think about an existing activity that you regularly use in your setting. How can you bring more structure to support children with ASD take turns as part of the activity?

### Outside equipment

I once worked with a specialist nursery setting (all ASD) where we set a great system to support turn taking for their outside play equipment. They put the following in place:

- A photo board with pictures of all of the equipment, including bikes, push carts, and so on, was posted.
- The children's pictures were matched to the equipment so that when they went outside, they were able to find their equipment.

## Social interaction

- Use of two-minute sand timers indicated how long each turn was. Staff used a five, four, three, two, one countdown.
- Staff consistently carried wait cards on their lanyards to offer a visual cue.
- There was consistent use of language around 'my turn', 'waiting', and 'finished'.
- Staff also had a short script they would read to the children around taking turns: 'Everyone will have a turn. I need to say my turn. I need to wait for my turn. I can watch the timer. Taking turns is a clever thing to do'.

Social interaction

## Social interaction activity sheet 8. Using a turn-taking board

**S:8**

This visual is helpful to use for children as part of a structured game with quick turns for children who understand 'wait'. Use of a wait card alongside the board would be helpful.

## Instructions for turn-taking board

- Copy the board (Figure 4.1) and laminate.
- Color in the borders of the top frame so it is green and cut it out before laminating so that it is clear in the middle.
- Color in the borders of the four bottom squares so they are red.
- Write the names or place a photo of who is in the group in a red square.
- Indicate whose turn it is by placing the green square over the top.

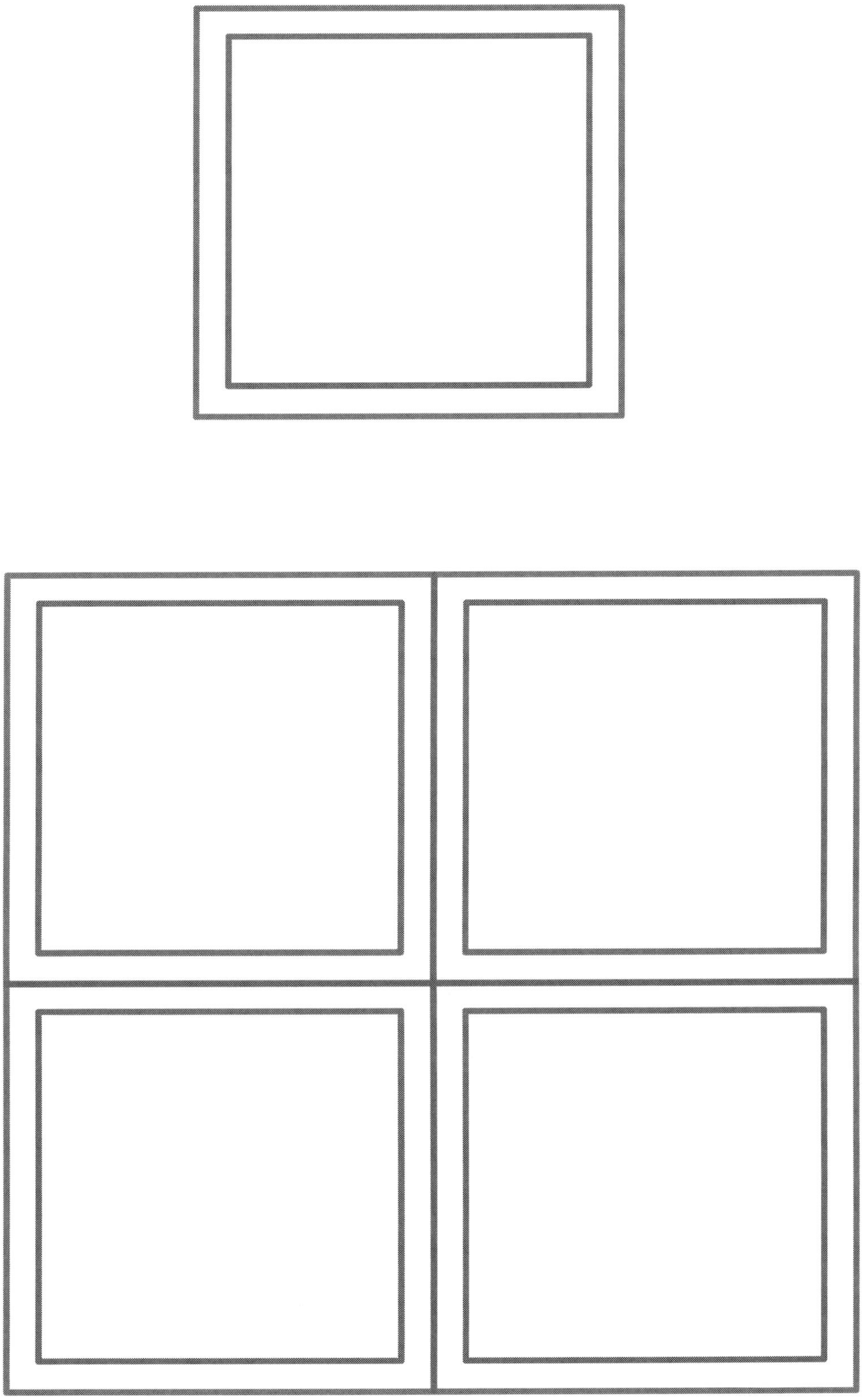

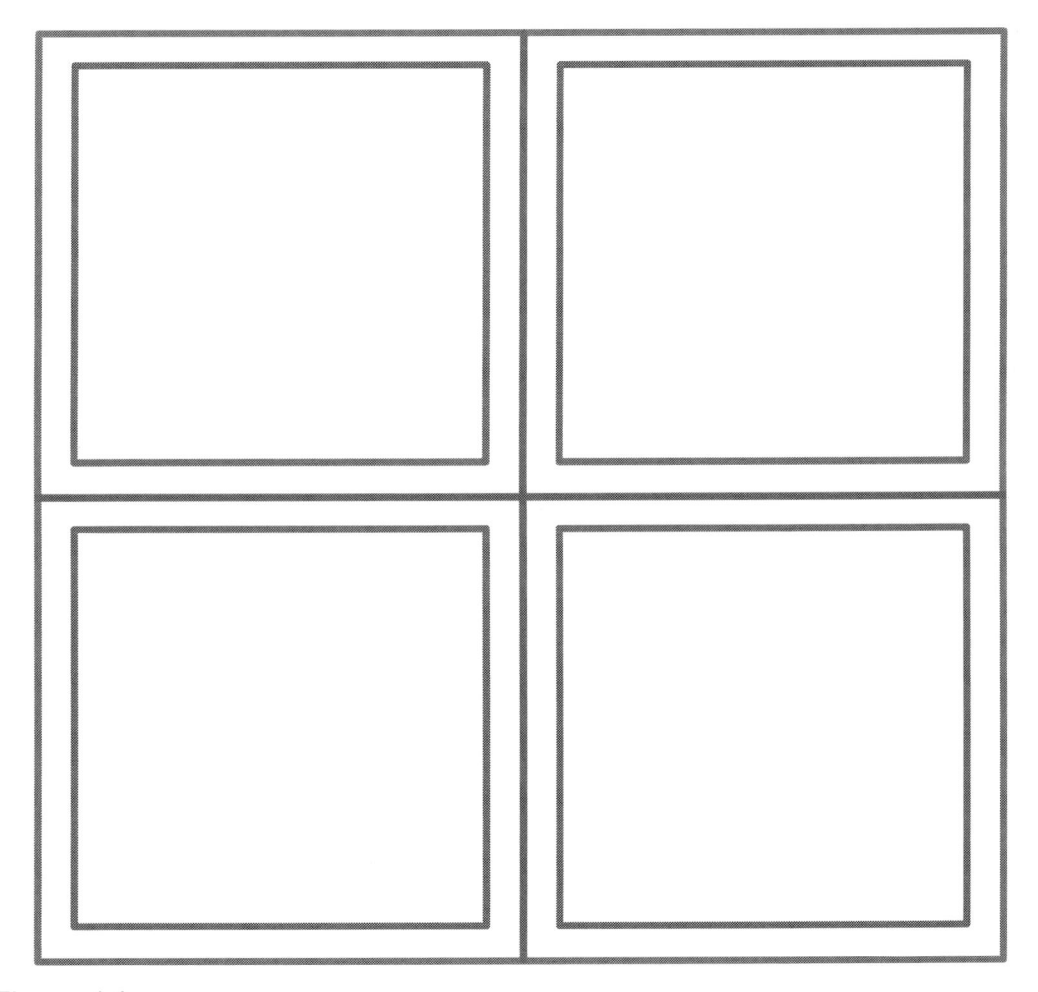

Figure 4.1

Social interaction

## Social interaction activity sheet 9.
## Let's chat – top tips for conversations

**S:9**

**We know that reciprocal social interaction is a key area of difficulty for children with ASD. Even for verbal children, conversation can be difficult because of the understanding of social cues required to be able to take turns and listen.**

**The following strategies provide some ideas for conversations for verbal children. There are many specific intervention programmes which seek to address conversation difficulties in children with ASD.**

### Get the conversation started

- Reduce your questions; instead, make comments.

- Offer conversational leads and pause; for example, instead of saying 'What did you do over the weekend?', say, 'Something funny happened to me over the weekend'.

- Build rapport by talking about a child's interests.

- Do something wrong on purpose as a funny way to start a conversation; for example, try to pour the juice with the lid on or say something incorrectly. If you know a child is good with colours, you could try labeling one incorrectly; wait to see if he or she corrects you.

- Use starter sentences: 'I like . . .' or 'My favourite is . . .'

- Give a context for conversations, for example, looking at a book or magazine, or adding social language (S5), such as 'I like it' or 'That is my favourite'.

### Use practical activities

- We know that when we provide a context, it is easier for children with ASD to engage. This makes the conversation less abstract.

- Use the child's about-me book (C16) as a context to start to start the conversation.

- Engage in a practical activity (C15) as a basis for conversation.

- Include other children in a practical activity; take photos of it and talk about it afterwards.

## Remember, you are the social guide

- Ensure that the experience is positive for a child with ASD to build confidence.
- As the adult, facilitate the child and repair the conversation if and when needed.
- Help the child build success.

Social interaction

## Social interaction activity sheet 10. Understanding others; foundations of theory of mind

**S:10**

In its simplest sense, theory of mind relates to the ability to understand the perspectives of others. From our knowledge of ASD, it is possible to see that this is an area of difficulty which has far-reaching consequences. Many intervention programmes seek to develop these skills. The approaches used tend to be suitable for older children. However, it is important to start developing the foundations of theory of mind in preschool children where possible.

- **Develop joint attention** – Earlier in this chapter we spoke about the links between joint attention and theory of mind. To understand others, a child needs to be able to pay attention to them.

- **A shared focus** – In (C1) we highlighted the importance for a shared focus, and throughout this manual we have emphasised the importance of this. We need this shared focus to develop the theory of mind a child needs to be able to pay attention to you. Use all the strategies discussed to establish a connection and rapport.

- **Encourage pretend play** – Chapter Five focusses in more detail on developing play skills in children with ASD. Pretend play presents many learning opportunities. By engaging in pretend play or especially role play, a child needs to take on a perspective of someone different.

- **Talk about feelings** – Make it clear why someone is feeling a particular way; for example, 'Oh, look, Sam is so happy', or 'She is really smiling because she likes that ice cream'. Put your child's feelings and your own into words; for example, 'I'm excited today, I am really looking forward to your school show'.

- **Talk about thoughts** – Start talking about the thoughts and feelings of characters and people this could be in relation to a television programme or a storybook. De Villiers and de Villiers (2014) highlight the importance of linking this back to the child. For example, if you are looking at a story in which a child is happy because it is his or her birthday, you could relate this to how the child with ASD felt on his or her birthday.

**Use books** – De Villiers and de Villiers (2014) highlight the importance of talking about characters; their thoughts, feelings, and actions; and what they may do next. As mentioned, it is also useful to relate this to the child.

**Think of others** – Talk about what other people may like to do or be interested in. For example, 'It is going to be Grandma's birthday' encourages a child with ASD to think about what Grandma would like.

## Materials needed

- None

## Chapter Four summary

- The social world can be a scary and overwhelming place for children with ASD.

- In the early years we can offer opportunities for positive social interaction and facilitate success. This doesn't always have to be turn taking and sharing; social success will depend on the individual child – for one child this may mean engaging in conversation; for another it may involve sharing eye contact and laughing.

- Just because children with ASD have social interaction difficulties doesn't mean they don't want to be social.

- We can use our knowledge of ASD to understand why social interaction is so difficult for children with ASD.

- Sensory difficulties can impact a child's ability to engage.

- Joint and shared attention are important skills to develop.

- By setting up a predictable environment (Chapter Two) and through providing consistent and appropriate support around communication (Chapter Three). we offer a good starting point to develop interaction.

## References

de Villiers, J. G. and de Villiers, P. A. (2014). The role of language in theory of mind development. *Topics in Language Disorders*, 34(4), 313–328.

Sussman, F. (2012). *More Than Words®: A Parent's Guide to Building Interaction and Language Skills for Children With Autism Spectrum Disorder or Social Communication Difficulties*. Toronto, Ontario: The Hanen Centre.

# Chapter Five
# PLAY SKILLS IN THE EARLY YEARS

**Chapter Five provides the following:**

- An overview of how play develops in typically developing children
- What the challenges are for children with ASD
- Top tips for supporting the development of play skills
- Activity sheets:

    **(P1) – Expanding a child's play interests**

    **(P2) – Sensory play activities**

    **(P3) – Ready, steady, go with play materials**

    **(P4) – Getting started with functional play**

    **(P5) – Let's pretend**

    **(P6) – Top toys for play**

## The importance of play

As adults working in the early years environment, you will be familiar with the philosophy that children learn a huge amount through play. Early years curriculums across the world have a shared philosophy around the importance of play.

Play is essentially a vehicle that allows children to develop a range of skills.

In typically developing children, play allows children to accomplish the following:

- Understand more about the world
- Develop motor skills

# Play skills in the early years

- Develop language
- Develop social interaction skills
- Develop problem-solving and thinking skills

Most children play naturally and do not need any prompting to do this. The rewards are part of the activity itself; children's natural curiosity leads them to experience different and new play activities.

When we are thinking about communication, it is important to be aware of the connection between play and language skills. Often, speech and language therapists stress the link between language and play skills; it is useful to understand a little more about this key connection and why it is important. When we pretend with a toy, we are using our symbolic comprehension; we need to understand that a cup can be a hat or that an apple can be a ball. This process of using something as something else involves symbolic thought. We need this for language development, as in the same way as an object represents something else, our words represent our thoughts. Although all play is important for a child's development, it is pretend play which is of key importance for communication skills.

When we consider the development of play, there are many different labels to describe similar levels and stages which can make the process of understanding play quite confusing. It is useful to look at some of the relevant theories related to play to provide an overview of what to expect in the children that you work with. Looking at what is typically expected is always helpful, as from there we can observe what a child with ASD is doing differently.

Tables 5.1 and 5.2 provide more information about the development of play.

Table 5.1 Parten's stages of play

| Age | Stage | Description |
| --- | --- | --- |
| Birth–3 months | **Unoccupied play** | At this stage babies are making a lot of movements with their arms, legs, hands, feet, etc. They are learning about and discovering how their bodies move. |
| Birth–2 years | **Solitary play** | This is the stage when children play alone. They are not interested in playing with others quite yet. |

| Age | Stage | Description |
|---|---|---|
| 2 years–2 ½ years | **Spectator/ onlooker** | During this stage a child begins to watch other children playing but does not play with them. |
| 2 ½ years–3 years | **Parallel play** | When a child plays alongside or near others but does not play with them, this stage is referred to as parallel play. |
| 3–4 years | **Associate play** | Children at this stage start to interact with others, but there may be only fleeting cooperation amongst them; for example, a child might be doing an activity related to those around him or her, but might not actually be interacting with another child. For example, they may all be playing on the same piece of playground equipment but all doing different things like climbing, swinging, etc. |
| 4 years and upwards | **Cooperative play** | When a child plays together with others and has interest in both the activity and other children involved in playing, they are participating in cooperative play. |

Adapted from Parten (1932)

Table 5.2 Different types of play activities (these are not presented as a developmental sequence; i.e., children do not have to complete them in a linear way)

| Type of play | Description |
|---|---|
| Exploratory | Babies and young children engage in exploratory play (sometimes also called sensorimotor play). Children are exploring their environment with their body and movements, banging, mouthing, and smelling. |
| Cause and effect | Cause-and-effect play occurs when children learn that they can make something happen by their actions, e.g., a pop-up toy or push-button object. |
| Functional | This is sometimes called relational play. Children understand the purpose of an object and can operate it in the appropriate way according to its function, e.g., pushing along a car or brushing their hair. |
| Pretend | Also known as symbolic play, an object is used for another purpose, e.g., holding a banana to your ear as a toy phone. |

The sixteen actions by sixteen months series produced by the FIRST WORDS PROJECT© on page 85 also provides an outline of play actions that a child will typically be engaged in.

## Play skills in children with ASD

Alongside delayed communication, difficulties with play are one of the first signs that parents realise their child is developing skills in a different way. Often parents contact me because their child is repetitive in their play or has an intense interest in a particular activity. Sometimes parents are concerned that their child may have an unusual focus on an item that is not a toy or they can focus on something for a very long time. These features can differentiate children from their typically developing peers.

I always imagine that this can be stressful at toddler groups when all the other children are exploring the activities and your child just wants to open and shut the door or lie down and look at all the wheels on the buggies. Of course, many typically developing children also do go through stages of this (but can generally be moved on quickly and they don't persist as an interest).

The play skills of children with ASD are affected by difficulties with social communication and interaction, reduced reciprocity (two-way communication), and also restricted and repetitive behaviours. This means that the play of children with ASD may lack flexibility, be repetitive, and have minimal social engagement. Going back to the stages of attention in Table 3.1, when children with ASD are single channelled, this may mean that they focus only on self-selected activities for long periods.

As mentioned, many typically developing children also go through stages of being repetitive in their play, for example, looking at items at eye level, lining up, opening and shutting things, and putting things into and out of containers. Part of this can be typical in terms of exploring the environment. When these activities become persistent or they become the only thing that a child will engage in, this can become difficult for a number of reasons, as it can then become challenging to move them onto different activities and for safety reasons.

In Chapter One we talked about gender differences in ASD. As highlighted by Imogen's insight in Chapter One, we need to understand how gender can impact the appearance of ASD in boys and girls. One area where these differences can be quite evident may be play skills. Research indicates the following relevant points are useful to be aware of when considering play skills of girls with ASD:

- Girls with ASD are often more aware of and feel a need to interact socially.
- Girls are involved in social play but often led by peers rather than initiating social contact.

- Girls are more socially inclined, and many have one special friend.

- Girls with ASD have more active imaginations and more often engage in pretend play than boys with ASD.

- Girls with ASD may also have interests that are more similar to their peers, for example, animals, books, favourite characters, and collectables. It is not the interests themselves that differentiate the girls; it is the intensity of these interests.

(Knickmeyer, Wheelwright, & Baron Cohen, 2008)

We know that children with ASD can find 'pretend' or 'symbolic' play difficult. This is not surprising, as pretend play relies on emerging theory of mind and the ability to use objects symbolically, both of which are challenging for children with ASD. We know from research that when children with ASD do engage in pretend play, it tends to be less sophisticated than their peers.

*Activity* Think about a child who you work with who has ASD. Consider the following key points.

- How do they play?

- What are they interested in?

- Does their play differ from other children who don't have ASD?

- What strengths in play have you observed?

- What areas of need have you observed in play?

Staff working with children with ASD often notice the following characteristics in the child's play (see Figure 5.1).

Given that play is such an important vehicle for development, it is important that we develop play skills alongside communication, interaction, and understanding.

Often when I see children engaging in the same activity again and again, I wonder if there is an additional reason behind this; in these cases I use the iceberg model to understand why this is happening (in Chapter Six we introduce the iceberg model as a tool for understanding behaviour). A child may be showing reduced and repetitive

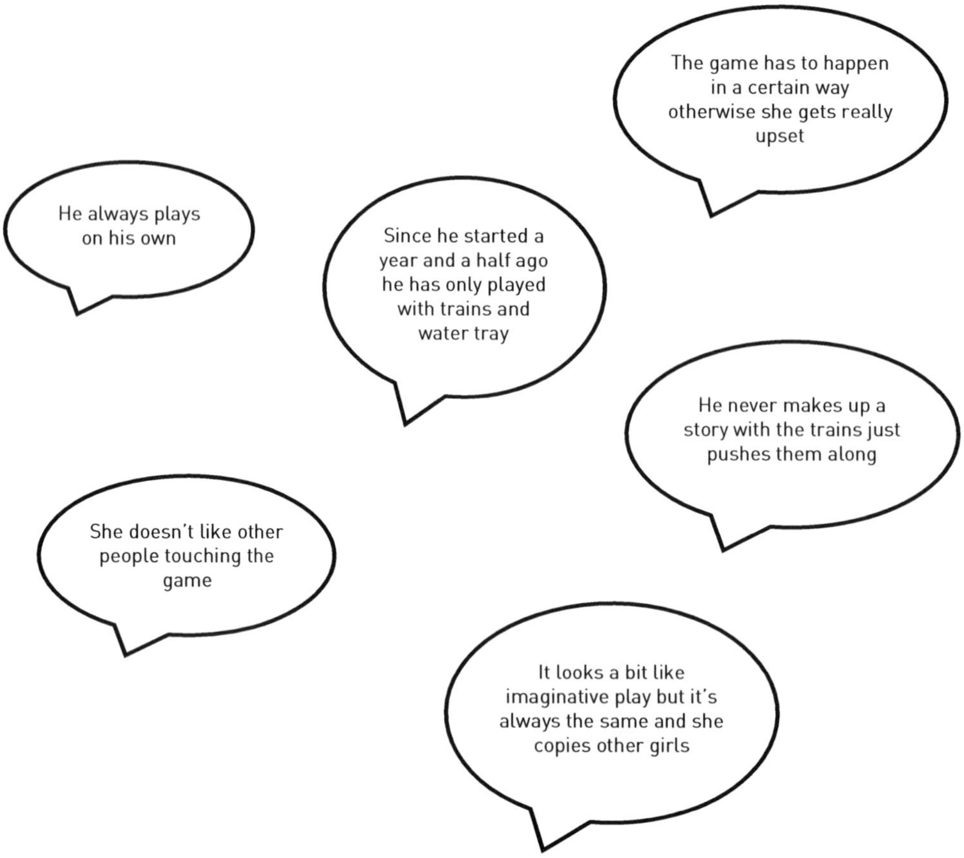

# Play skills in the early years

> He always plays on his own

> Since he started a year and a half ago he has only played with trains and water tray

> The game has to happen in a certain way otherwise she gets really upset

> He never makes up a story with the trains just pushes them along

> She doesn't like other people touching the game

> It looks a bit like imaginative play but it's always the same and she copies other girls

Figure 5.1

behaviour for a number of reasons. Commonly observed reasons include the following:

- **A lack of play skills** – A child with ASD often isn't sure of what else to do. Even in an education environment full of toys, they are unsure of what to do and how to play with them.

- **A repetitive behaviour that makes a child feel safe and secure** – In Chapter Two we discussed how important the environment and structure can be in reducing anxiety and promoting independence. When a child with ASD is unsure of the routine and what is happening, repetitive behaviours can increase. Optimising the environment as discussed in Chapter Two can have a big impact on a range of skills.

- **A sensory need** – Some children show behaviours that are fulfilling a sensory need. Often this may be persistent throwing or climbing. In these cases (usually when the behaviour is significant and impacting on the child's ability to engage in anything else) advice from an OT can be helpful.

## Top tips for play

By now you should be familiar with the following strategies as they have been emphasised in all the previous chapters. It is useful to recap them to ensure you keep them in mind when playing.

- Be at the child's level.
- Follow their interests.
- Develop a connection.
- Don't impose your agenda or ask repeated questions.
- Gradually introduce new elements to the game.
- Provide opportunities for repetition across contexts.

## When play becomes challenging and difficult to manage

**TIP** We focus on behaviour that challenges in more detail in the next chapter. However, it is important to mention here as well that sometimes a play action can become difficult to manage or pose a risk to the child or others in the environment; for example, opening and shutting doors or constant climbing can become dangerous. On these occasions you need to be a detective and look for the underlying reason as to why this is occurring (this is discussed in more detail in Chapter Six). It may be that if a play action such as opening or shutting doors has a repetitive component and it is difficult to re-focus a child, there could be a sensory component to the action. If the action is interfering with the child's ability to engage in other activities, then it might be useful to consider a referral to OT. It may be that in some cases you can offer a safer alternative as a compromise; for example, for children who throw everything, give them opportunities for appropriate throwing, for example, tossing bean bags into a box. I worked with a child who had a dangerous obsession with opening and shutting doors so much so that he opened the oven. He was given a small doll's wardrobe to open and shut, and at times this was a distraction and reduced the opening and shutting of actual doors.

We turn now to the activity sheets as part of this chapter. These provide a range of activities and strategies to support the development of play skills.

Just remember, play has to be fun!

Play skills in the early years

## Play activity sheet 1. Expanding a child's play interests

**P:1**

**Children with ASD can be repetitive in their play. This can mean that they tend to stick to certain activities or sequences of play. I remember seeing a little boy in a nursery who had attended for over two and a half years; when I asked them what he played with, they responded that he had only ever played with cars and trains and had never engaged with anything else.**

**Even if a child is not ready for pretending, we can expand the range of other types of play they engage in, for example, exploratory, cause and effect, and functional.**

**When children are self-directed in their play, you can join alongside and start imitating them (C3). It can be useful for you to have the same materials so that you are not directly imposing on what they are doing; instead you are playing alongside.**

## Use an interest to learn a new skill

Using children's interests is a good way to get them to extend what they are doing and play with other things. Be creative in your planning, and encourage a child to try new and different activities. Remember, it needs to be fun!

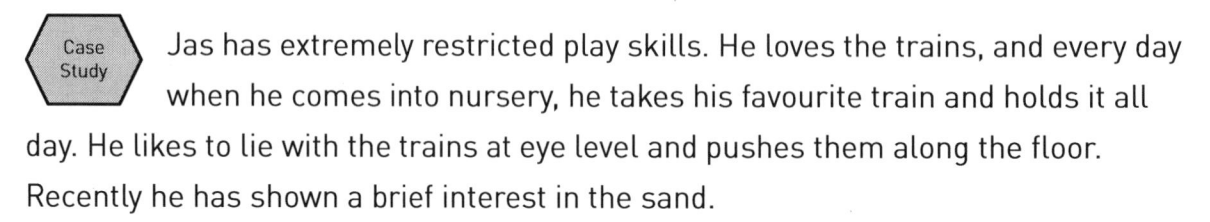

*Case Study* — Jas has extremely restricted play skills. He loves the trains, and every day when he comes into nursery, he takes his favourite train and holds it all day. He likes to lie with the trains at eye level and pushes them along the floor. Recently he has shown a brief interest in the sand.

Staff working with Jas started to incorporate his interest into other activities to try and expand his play. They focussed on the following activities:

- Driving trains and cars through sand and other materials, for example, lentils and rice

- Using different types of cars and vehicles (Jas tends to prefer small, metal cars and loves Thomas the Tank Engine) – they have introduced a fire engine alongside some wooden cars

- Introducing the garage

# Play skills in the early years

- Pushing the car down the ramp as part of a ready, steady, go game
- Using Jas's interest in Thomas the Tank Engine to introduce some Thomas the Tank Engine books and colouring sheets

## Materials needed

- Tailored to the child's interests

Play skills in the early years

## Play activity sheet 2.
## Sensory play activities

**P:2**

For some children who are at the early stages of play, the toys and activities as part of the nursery environment may not be motivating. I saw a child recently where the staff who were in tune with the child had noticed that he wasn't interested in anything. He would walk around and fleetingly stay at a table. They adapted the play materials in the environment and provided a great opportunity for joint and shared attention and a shared social experience. Not all settings have the luxury of a sensory room. Try and use some of these simple activity ideas to create a space for a child with ASD to explore.

**Use of a tent or quiet calming area** – A tent can offer a quiet space for a child with ASD. If you don't have one, be creative and make a calming area. Go back to (E9) and (E10) to think about how the environment is structured.

**Glittery water bottle** – Add water, glitter, and food colouring to a clear, two-litre bottle. Add some strong tape around the lid to ensure that there are no spills.

**Messy play** – Try shaving foam or corn flour with water. Add colours and glitter, or encourage a child to get involved by including a favourite toy; for example, walk a dinosaur through it.

**Coloured spaghetti** – You can create different-coloured spaghetti. In my experience children love this, and it can be fun to explore, plus there is no need to worry if it ends up being eaten.

- Cook spaghetti as usual.
- In a sealable bag, add vegetable oil and food colouring.
- Add the spaghetti to the bag and leave it for fifteen minutes.
- Rinse excess colour from the spaghetti in cold water.

**Moon sand** – If you aren't familiar with moon sand, it is a great texture to mould, sieve, and drive things through. It is easy and quick to make.

- Mix eight cups of flour and one cup of baby oil.
- I have added different smells, as this can be interesting for some children to explore.

**Bubble wrap popping** – Walking or rolling on bubble wrap can be highly motivating and a great way to explore new textures and sounds.

**Tinfoil blanket** – This is one of my top therapy materials – they are inexpensive and can instantly transfer into an activity, for example, peekaboo, hiding, or pouring lentils onto it.

## Materials needed

- Dependent on the child's interests

*Play skills in the early years*

## Play activity sheet 3.
## Ready, steady, go with play materials

**P:3**

We have talked about how we can use ready, steady, go games to develop communication and interaction skills. We can also use them to encourage a child to engage in a range of play activities. Ready, steady, go is essentially a cause-and-effect type activity as when the child sends you a message for 'go', he or she is making something happen.

**Use ready, steady, go games in the following activities.**

# Pouring

Pouring can be visually appealing and motivating to children with ASD. It doesn't have to be water; rice and lentils also make a great sound. Try pouring these materials:

- Sand
- Water (you could add food colouring)
- Rice
- Lentils

# Shaking

Be creative; think about what a child is interested in. These all lend themselves to a stop/go game as outlined in (C8).

Try shaking these:

- A tinfoil blanket
- A tray of rice or lentils
- Shakers and other instruments
- Sifting flour onto black paper (this is from the Attention Autism programme by Gina Davies)

# Auditory

These can also be uses as part of a stop/go game:

- Playing music with an on/off switch
- Banging on drums
- Crinkling a tinfoil blanket

## Play activity sheet 4.
## Getting started with functional play

**P:4**

When we talk about functional play, we are referring to an action in which a child is demonstrating the function. This could be a wide range of activities. I often observe that children with ASD will show some functional play but can get stuck in the same action or type of action, for example, playing with vehicles.

**Try these simple activities to get a child to start or expand functional play skills.**

When children start engaging in more functional play activities, it can be a great time to build on this. Children at this stage may be quite self-directed and have limited attention, so it is useful to be able to use these strategies across the day rather than feeling that you need to sit down and specifically target them.

- **Introduce a favourite toy or puppet into your daily activities** – Sit the toy at the snack table and model 'I think teddy is hungry'. Encourage the child to feed him by using gestures (rubbing your tummy and saying 'Mmmm') and also pointing to the toy. Having a doll whose hands you can wash can be helpful. Involve the toy in different functional activities across the day.

- **Think of the child's interests** – For a child who looks at a car at eye level and spins the wheels, incorporate a ramp where you can 'whoosh' the car down. Or for a child who likes to line up bricks, use hand over hand to help him or her make a tower and 'crash' or knock it down.

- **Link interests to play** – I worked with a girl who was interested in lining up bottles. She would spend a long time lining up any bottle or container in different shapes and then knock them all down. We introduced a domino game, and this replaced the bottles. She was motivated by the pattern and way that the bottles fell, which was why dominos were so interesting for her.

- **Imitate and add something new** – If children who you work with are repetitive in their play, for example, opening and shutting the door on the toy oven or spinning the wheels on a car, they may become absorbed in this. You could join them with your own toy and then copy their actions; we know from (C3) that copying can help a child pay attention to us. Once we have the child's attention, we can do something practical, such as place the car on the ground, push it along, and say 'Brum, brum'.

## Play activity sheet 5. Let's pretend

**P:5**

**Through closely observing the play skills of a child who you work with, you will have built up a picture of his or her skills and abilities. Think of these in terms of the stages of play and also the different types of play (as described in Tables 5.1 and 5.2 earlier in this chapter). If children are demonstrating functional play (using items as intended), for example, brushing their hair with a brush or putting a toy phone to their ear, you can introduce the following play activities to extend these skills.**

- **Have one of your own** – If the child that you are playing with is focussed on a doll or a teddy, ensure that you also have one. This means that you can imitate what the child is doing and also add your own play actions.

- **Add to the sequence** – If a child carries out simple functional activities, for example, feeding the teddy a bottle, you can add to the sequence to help the child extend play. For example, after the teddy has had a bottle, say 'Teddy's tired', and hold out the cover to see if the child will cover up the teddy. You could then add another action and say 'Night, night', and give the teddy a kiss. Remember not to direct the child or tell him or her to 'Say good night to teddy'. Offer opportunities and remember to pause (C2).

- **Add different objects** – If a child already has functional play where he or she is using a realistic object for its intended purpose, for example, holding a toy phone to the ear, you can add to this by using different play actions such as pretending to hold an imaginary phone or holding a banana as a phone.

- **Include other children when you pretend** – This has the advantage of laying the foundations of cooperative play. You can also use the other children as models. If you pretend that a blanket is a spaceship, you can ask who is going to be an astronaut and who will be an alien.

- **Add a new action** – For example, if a child pours a pretend cup of tea, you can pretend to spill it! By doing something unexpected, you are providing a cue for the child to think of what comes next. If he or she doesn't naturally do this, you can offer a cue; for example, hold out a tissue for him or her to wipe up the tea.

**Provide variation** – Often I see children who will show some pretend play actions, but they tend to be fairly limited and restricted, for example, making a cup of tea and pretending it's hot. Try to model a range of play actions, and be inventive about what you are doing.

**Use props in the environment** – Most early years settings have a home corner with a kitchen or dressing up area; using hats can be a great way to start this. Many children with ASD who I have worked with have found dressing up and role play difficult. It is important to bear this in mind and go at the child's pace. Also through tailoring it to their interests, you are more likely to get a positive response.

## Play activity sheet 6.
## Top toys for play

P:6

**There are so many toys available to purchase and also so many 'educational' toys available that sometimes we can lose sight that often the simplest toys are the best. First and foremost, *you* are the best toy; the opportunities that you can offer as a play partner and in facilitating interaction outweigh many other activities. People often ask me about useful toys. Here is a general list of inexpensive and easy-to-use activities.**

- **A large tray for messy play** – This has the added advantage of providing a clear visual cue to the child as to what the activity is. You could use a certain space in the environment to provide consistency and increase the physical structure in the environment.

- **Bubbles** – They can be used in so many ways.

- **A puppet, preferably with a noisemaker and a mouth that moves** – This can be much more motivating than a doll to get children with ASD interested in functional play, such as feeding, brushing, and so on.

- **Vehicles that don't have logos** – They can be used for different things, for example, a plain car, boat, and lorry. You can develop pretend skills by adding meaning to the objects, for example, 'It's a speed boat', or pretending the lorry is an ambulance.

- **Small bag of functional play materials to use with the puppet** – Try a toothbrush, hair brush, blanket, and spoon.

- **Parachute**

- **Scarves for playing peekaboo** – Scarves that can be seen through work well.

- **Several sensory cause-and-effect toys** – Depending on the individual child, you will want to tailor these to their preferences, for example, auditory, visual, or movement.

- **Plastic containers with lids**

- **Dried rice or lentils**

- **Food colouring**

- **Cardboard boxes** – These are invaluable to use as part of pretend play; for example, make it into a shop, a boat, and so on.

- **Hats** – They are less threatening than a full fancy dress costume, but still encourage a child with ASD to take on a different role.

## Materials needed

- Ideas as listed
- It can be useful to go back to the Skills Profile and consider where a child is in terms of all their skills

## Chapter Five summary

- Play is a fundamental part of child development. Children learn new skills through play.

- Play skills in children with ASD can develop in a different way due to difficulties with two-way communication, restricted and repetitive behaviours, and self-directed attention.

- Pretend play is important for language.

- Girls with ASD may be more adept at play. Their play skills may be more similar to typically developing peers.

## References

Knickmeyer, R. C., Wheelwright, S. and Baron-Cohen, S. B. (2008). Sex-typical play: Masculinization/defeminization in girls with an autism spectrum condition. *Journal of Autism and Developmental Disorders*, 38(6), 1028–1035.

Parten, M. B. (1932). Social participation among preschool children. *Journal of Abnormal and Social Psychology*, 27(3), 243–269.

# Chapter Six
# MAKING SENSE OF BEHAVIOUR

> **Chapter Six provides the following:**
>
> - An overview of behaviour – the clinical psychologist perspective
> - An emphasis on being a detective and helping you use all the tools and knowledge you have gathered on ASD
> - Introduction to the iceberg model
> - ABC charts
> - Prevention and preparation
> - Top tips for managing behaviour
> - Strategy sheets
> - Activity sheets:
>
>   **(B1) – The iceberg model**
>
>   **(B2) – ABC chart**
>
>   **(B3) – Pull it together - let's make a behaviour plan**
>
>   **(B4) – 'I am working for'**

## You may ask why is there a chapter on behaviour in a book about communication

Good question!

In my work with children with ASD, I have often been saddened by number of failed school placements and difficulties children with ASD face in the education environment. Often 'behaviour' is cited as the reason. The statistics on school exclusion for children

## Making sense of behaviour

with ASD are high; the sad reality is that children with ASD who are already facing challenges can't even access the support they need, thus leaving them disadvantaged.

In the early years we can help understand behaviour and understand why a child may be behaving a certain way. In many cases, behaviour is a form of communication and is usually telling us something. As we understand the communication, we can also make sense of the behaviour.

I have learnt a lot from the wonderful clinical psychologists I have worked with who have taught me that rather than jumping in and looking immediately for a solution to a problem, we need to delve deeper and attempt to understand why the behaviour is occurring in the first place. Without this understanding, we will never reach the reason for the behaviour.

## An introduction to behaviour that challenges

Dr Rachel McCarthy, clinical psychologist, provides an overview.

Behaviour that challenges such as pushing, hitting, and biting can be common in all children at a certain age and stage, but it is generally expected that as a child develops communication and social skills, such as learning to share, wait, and turn take, such behaviours will gradually subside.

When behaviours do not subside, it generally causes concern, and carers are keen to stop the behaviours. This often leads to strategies being put in place before the underlying cause of the behaviour is fully understood, meaning that the chances of the strategies working are reduced.

## Making sense of behaviour – be a detective

- Making sense of the behaviour first is important, and we often use the analogy of being a 'detective'.
- This means looking closely at the behaviour, including what happened just before the behaviour occurred and what happened afterwards.
- ABC charts are a useful way of collecting this information; see (B2) for an example of an ABC chart.
- In an ABC chart, A stands for 'antecedent', which essentially means 'trigger' – that is, what triggered the behaviour?

- The B stands for the 'behaviour' itself that you saw; it is helpful to describe the behaviour rather than label it. For example, 'Jack picked up a beaker and hit Zoe over the head with it' rather than 'Jack was naughty'.

- The C stands for 'consequences', which means looking at what happened immediately after the behaviour. For example, after Jack hit Zoe on the head with the beaker, his key worker rushed over, picked him up, and carried him away.

- Keeping detailed ABC charts for up to a week can help get a really good understanding of the frequency of the behaviours, the triggers to the behaviours, and a sense of what factors may be reinforcing the behaviour.

Playing the detective is important because the reason for one child hitting is unlikely to be the same as another child hitting.

In this chapter you will be introduced to another helpful model for making sense of behaviour – the iceberg model. Having a reasonable understanding of why a child is behaving in a certain way will be far more likely to lead to appropriate solutions and strategies in the long run. Remember, one size does not fit all!

Although behaviour that challenges can be frustrating and sometimes distressing for those around the child, it is important to remember that all behaviour has a function and is meaningful for the individual, even if it is not immediately apparent what this meaning is. Using ABC charts and the iceberg model, along with all the information and knowledge you have now acquired about ASD, will help you help the child.

## The iceberg model

Many approaches use the analogy of an iceberg to help understand behaviour. This is a great visual way to understand what may be going on for a child with ASD. Using the iceberg can be useful for any child showing a behaviour that you want to problem solve. The key thing is that it helps us to look at the 'why'.

Most of the iceberg is hidden under the water, and we see only the top. This part is the behaviour. The majority is hidden under the water, and this is the reason as to why it is happening.

Sometimes when we just look at the top of the iceberg we fail to see what is going on underneath (see Figure 6.1). Without understanding why a behaviour is occurring, we are unable to provide a strategy that works.

## Making sense of behaviour

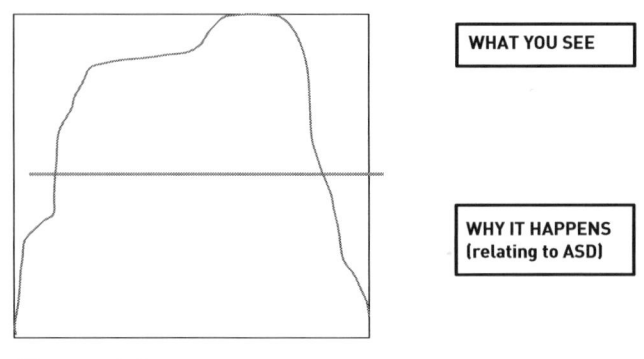

Figure 6.1

[WHAT YOU SEE]

[WHY IT HAPPENS (relating to ASD)]

For example, if we focus on the visible behaviours on the top of the iceberg, such as hitting, biting, throwing, pushing, and spitting, we don't see the underlying factors related to the child's diagnosis of ASD. These could include that a child with ASD is unaware of social rules, has sensory sensitivities, is frustrated, is attempting to communicate, is unaware of the feelings of others, or is unaware of a more appropriate social response. The 'why' will vary depending on each child and situation. Often when we think about behaviour that challenges, the first thing that comes to mind is aggressive behaviours such as those just mentioned. Often children with ASD show behaviours that aren't necessarily challenging, but it is still important to understand why they are occurring. Some commonly observed behaviours that aren't aggressive but can still be challenging may include the child being passive; some people may feel that the child is being lazy and is reliant on adult prompts and lacking independence. For a child who presents like this, the following factors may be going on underneath the iceberg; the child is unaware of expectations, is not motivated by typical rewards, has a poor concept of time, or doesn't understand future rewards.

See (B1) for a copy of the iceberg model that you can photocopy and use in your setting. Use the iceberg to look at the behaviour (the part you can see) and what is going on underneath in terms of the ASD (the part you can't see).

**TIP** Take time to understand the 'why'. Talk to the parents; get their thoughts. Gather information, and as Dr McCarthy suggests, *be a detective*. All too often we are keen to rush in and try different strategies before fully understanding what the problems are. However, the time you spend is invaluable and will contribute to a far greater understanding of the issues and why they are happening, which ultimately leads you to a more effective solution.

The following case study about Jack and Ahmed highlights the importance in gathering the correct information so that you can really understand *why* a particular

# Making sense of behaviour

behaviour may be occurring. Without the 'why', it is difficult to put in place an effective strategy.

> **Case Study**
>
> **Behaviour observed: hitting**
>
> Jack and Ahmed attend the same early years setting. They both have a diagnosis of ASD and are often observed to be hitting different children. Staff have decided as a group to be consistent, say 'No hitting', and remove Jack or Ahmed from the situation when they hit.

Unfortunately the strategy isn't working, and both children continue to hit other children. The behaviours are escalating, and other parents are commenting on both Jack and Ahmed hitting their children.

On the advice of an SLT, staff decided to use the iceberg model and use an ABC chart as a way to gather more information about the behaviour.

### Jack's iceberg

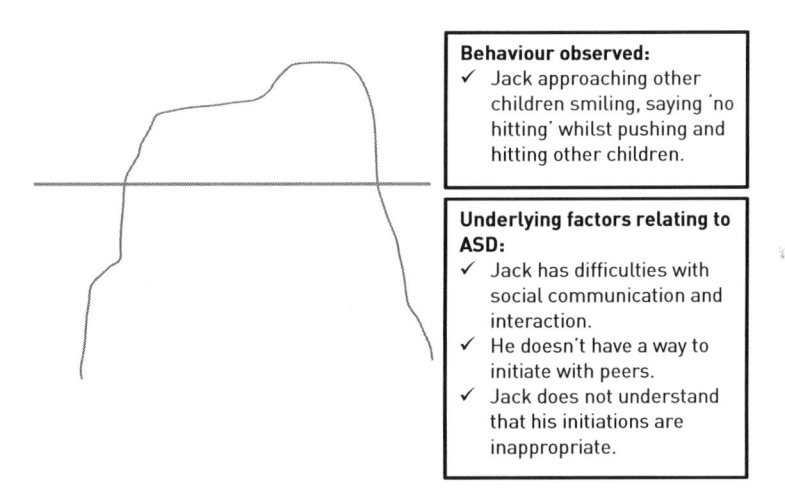

**Behaviour observed:**
- ✓ Jack approaching other children smiling, saying 'no hitting' whilst pushing and hitting other children.

**Underlying factors relating to ASD:**
- ✓ Jack has difficulties with social communication and interaction.
- ✓ He doesn't have a way to initiate with peers.
- ✓ Jack does not understand that his initiations are inappropriate.

Staff working with Jack kept an ABC chart. From their observations they were able to conclude that Jack was using his behaviour as a way to communicate and interact.

### What happened next?

- Staff working with Jack focussed on teaching him appropriate ways to engage with peers.
- Instead of just saying 'No hitting', they focussed on teaching him alternative behaviours to replace the hitting. They modelled 'gentle hands' and used helpful social phrases: 'Can I play?', 'Chase me', and 'My turn'.
- Staff also included Jack in a small social group with a focus on providing a positive shared social experience, turn taking, and social language.

## Ahmed's iceberg

**AHMED'S ICEBERG**

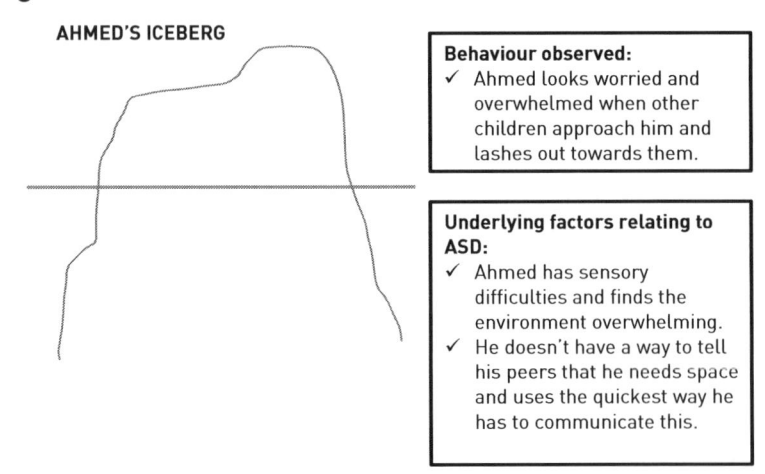

**Behaviour observed:**
- ✓ Ahmed looks worried and overwhelmed when other children approach him and lashes out towards them.

**Underlying factors relating to ASD:**
- ✓ Ahmed has sensory difficulties and finds the environment overwhelming.
- ✓ He doesn't have a way to tell his peers that he needs space and uses the quickest way he has to communicate this.

Staff also completed an ABC chart for Ahmed, a segment of which is detailed in Table 6.1.

Table 6.1 Ahmed's ABC chart

| Date/time/place | Antecedent | Behaviour | Consequence | Other observations |
|---|---|---|---|---|
| 18.10.2019 | Ahmed is in the queue waiting for his lunch. He appears quite overwhelmed. | Ahmed screamed and pushed another child on the shoulder. | Ahmed removed from the queue and taken to a quiet space. | Ahmed seemed tired and a little anxious about the noise and smell of lunch. |

From their detective work with the iceberg and the ABC chart, staff concluded that Ahmed found it difficult to cope at transition times. He found unstructured times between activities stressful. Ahmed is easily overwhelmed by the environment and wants to leave the situation. He has no way to tell anyone this. Using his behaviour to communicate is a quick and successful way to get himself out of a stressful situation.

### What happened next?

- Staff working with Ahmed focussed on giving him a clear way to communicate 'no' or that he wanted to leave a situation; they effectively replaced the hitting behaviour with a communicative behaviour.

- Staff also helped reduce Ahmed's anxiety around transitions by increasing structure and using a portable visual timetable and first/then board; they also timetabled in more 'quiet time'.

- Collectively, these strategies saw an elimination of the hitting behaviours.

**Case Study:** Jemima is four and a half. She is an articulate girl, and staff working with her report that she copes well in the early years environment. Occasionally she has a meltdown, and staff can't understand why this happens. When this happens Jemima is distressed, and she is unable to explain why she is upset.

Staff working with Jemima kept an ABC chart over several weeks and worked out that the meltdowns occured when there were cut flowers in the reception area of the nursery.

Staff talked to Jemima's mum, and she explained that Jemima is extremely sensitive to certain smells.

This case study highlights the impact that sensory factors can have on children with ASD. (I remember once talking to an adult with ASD who explained that the sound of wiping kitchen surfaces felt like it was 'cutting his ears'.)

**Case Study:** Leon is three years and ten months. He has a diagnosis of ASD. He has a few words that he uses. He has responded well to support from staff working with him focussing on copying his vocalisations and developing interactive games. Leon has recently started to bite staff hard on the shoulder. Staff feel that the behaviour comes from nowhere, and Leon often laughs when he is doing it. Staff are understandably upset by this behaviour and are thinking about whether they should use time out.

To gather more information about where this behaviour is coming from, staff kept an ABC chart for ten days.

### Leon's iceberg

From their detective work with the iceberg and the ABC chart (Table 6.2), staff started to notice a pattern of when Leon would bite. It always tended to be after an enjoyable activity when he was excited. The adult response 'cross face and change of voice' was quite motivating for Leon and reinforced the biting; essentially he enjoyed what happened as a consequence to his biting and continued to do it. Through completing the ABC chart, staff also picked up on a wider range of sensory needs.

## Making sense of behaviour

**Behaviour observed:**
- ✓ Leon smiles, looks at adult and bites them on the shoulder after an interactive game.

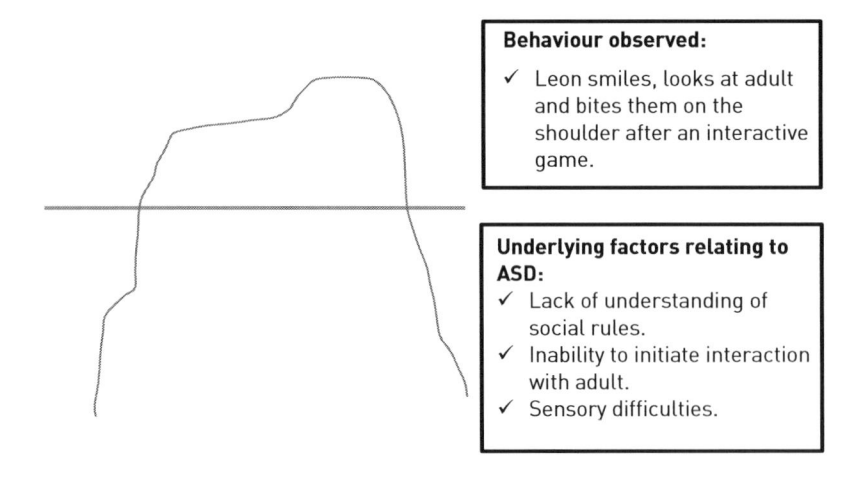

**Underlying factors relating to ASD:**
- ✓ Lack of understanding of social rules.
- ✓ Inability to initiate interaction with adult.
- ✓ Sensory difficulties.

Table 6.2 Leon's ABC chart

| Date/time/place | Antecedent | Behaviour | Consequence | Other observations |
|---|---|---|---|---|
| 5.10.2017 | Leon has been enjoying a tickling game with a member of staff. | Leon looks at the member of staff, leans over her back, and bites her shoulder, laughing. | Staff working with Leon say 'No biting, Leon, stop', accompanied with a cross facial expression. | Leon does not seem to understand what they are telling him and continues to laugh. |

**What happened next?**

- Staff met with Leon's parents to see if biting was happening at home, wrote a behaviour plan, and established a consistent response to when he bit.

- Staff agreed to all respond in a consistent yet neutral way, saying 'Stop' in a calm voice and moving Leon away and onto a different activity with a neutral facial expression.

- Alongside this they focussed on teaching Leon more appropriate initiations for interaction, including using songs and people games.

- Leon was also referred to OT as there seemed to be a sensory component to his biting (he also mouthed a lot of other toys).

- As a result, over a period of eight weeks, the biting reduced.

This example highlights that behaviour doesn't change quickly. Consistency is key in managing behaviour, and it's important to stick with strategies before feeling that they aren't working.

# Making sense of behaviour

**TIP** Look after yourself. This may sound silly, but being bitten, hit, or spat at is not fun, even when it is a small person, and it can be upsetting. Make sure you talk it through with someone, step away from the situation, and have a break and a drink. Being bitten can especially leave you feeling shaken. Remember, if a bite breaks the skin, you may need to follow up with your general practitioner. Always follow your setting's policy on reporting incidents.

**Activity** Think of a child who you work with or have worked with who has a diagnosis of ASD; were there ever behaviours that you were unsure as to why they occurred? Draw out an iceberg, and be a detective to try and discover why these occurred.

## Reinforcing behaviours

In these case studies we briefly talked about 'reinforcing behaviours'. What do we mean by this? Reinforcement is how a behaviour is strengthened by what happens after it as a consequence. In other words, if you behave in a certain way and this gets what you want, you are more likely to continue to engage in the same behaviour again and again when you want the same thing to happen.

In Ahmed's example when he hit another child, he was quickly removed from the situation, giving him some quiet time, which is what he wanted. You can see how this then reinforced the behaviour of hitting. Similarly for Leon, he was highly motivated by making an adult's face change and viewed this as a continuation of the interaction he was enjoying; the adult response reinforced the behaviour, and he consequently continued to bite as it had become motivating to him.

This is one of the reasons why time out doesn't work for children with ASD. Often a child may need a break, so removing him or her from the situation as a result of a behaviour is essentially reinforcing the behaviour.

We can use positive reinforcement to encourage positive behaviours. Reinforcement is the opposite of punishment as it aims to increase a behaviour rather than decrease it. We incentivise and reward all children, for example by giving them stars on a chart and praise for using the toilet as opposed to taking away a privilege for not using the toilet. Many of the approaches that we have covered use rewards and positive reinforcement, for example, first/then boards.

Think about the reinforcement that you are offering a child and whether it is meaningful to him or her. I remember an adult speaker with ASD telling the group, 'Of course she wasn't going to do complete tasks when her teacher said that by doing the work, it would make Miss Smith really happy and proud, but if they said complete your work for ten minutes on the trampoline, she would do it straightaway'. The premise of this is similar to the 'I am working for' board in (B3).

When you are being a detective, you need to consider all factors relating to ASD that may be affecting a child and how he or she communicates and behaves. Remember, you can use the iceberg model as a tool to help you understand a range of behaviours, not just those that are challenging.

As we mentioned earlier, behaviour that challenges can be stressful for all involved. One of the major things that can be done to support behaviours is prevention. Being prepared is of key importance.

## Preparation

In many cases I have gone into an early years setting where staff are surprised by the level of need or difficulty a child may be having. The child has started at the setting, and the staff have had little or no prior warning that the child may have additional needs.

In Chapter One I mentioned that some of the most successful placements for young children with ASD haven't necessarily been a result of vast experience but a result of good preparation, an open mind, and careful planning.

If you know that you have a child arriving in your setting, you can prepare for their arrival; this will make the process much smoother for them and for you.

> **TIP** Use the preparation checklist below to help you prepare for a child with ASD.

## Preparation checklist

- If possible, try to do a home visit before the child starts. This gives the advantage of seeing a child in his or her own surroundings where he or she will likely be most confident and communicate naturally.

- Complete the Skills Profile as a baseline measure.

- Think about the physical environment; go back to (E9).

- Do all staff have some understanding of ASD? Dispel stereotypes and misinformation by completing the quiz in Chapter One.

- Complete the Skills Profile and Information-Gathering Tool with parents prior to a child starting so that you have as much information as possible before they start.

## Prevention is key

**Activity** — Think about your setting. Use your knowledge of ASD to help you address potential problem areas for the children you work with. By now you have a good understanding of the core difficulties of ASD and how different children may experience these.

Instead of thinking 'This is how I will stop *this behaviour*', brainstorm how you will adapt your environment and yourself to minimise the chance of behaviours occurring in the first place.

**TIP** — Don't miss out on the 'why'. Sometimes when we become familiar with a child and understand lots about ASD, it is quite easy to jump straight to using a strategy without taking time to understand the 'why'. It is always a worthwhile exercise to complete an iceberg or an ABC chart.

Remember that behaviour may show in different contexts. I have worked with some children who do not show any behaviour that challenges at all at school, but home is a different picture. Often children who are relatively able manage to hold it together all day only to have meltdowns afterwards. Becky, who shared her parental perspective of having a child with ASD in Chapter One, was a similar picture to this.

## Teaching a replacement

I once worked with a teacher whose golden rule around behaviour was 'don't say no, say ohhhh'; the oh part is to have a chance to think about how to respond. Think of how often we are saying 'no' to children with ASD. Instead of just saying no as in 'No hitting' with Jack and Ahmed, we need to think what behaviour we want the child to be doing instead and teaching them this.

> **TIP** Tell a child what to do, not what not to do. This is a powerful and helpful strategy that most people are familiar with when supporting behaviour. If you have children running down a corridor and the adult is shouting 'No running', in essence the children hear 'running' and keep going. Instead, if the adults say 'Walking', they are telling the child clearly and directly what they are expected to be doing.

## Top tips for supporting behaviour

- **Understand ASD** – The ability to get into the shoes of children with ASD will help you in your ability to problem solve what is happening for them. Remember Imogen in Chapter One? By understanding ASD we effectively put ourselves in the child's shoes. This way we can see the world from their perspective and adapt what we are doing accordingly.

- **Analyse the behaviour** – Use the tools that you have learnt in this chapter: (B1) and (B2).

- **Adapt the environment** – We know from Chapter Two and the insight into the TEACCH® approach that if we can bring structure to the environment, we can promote independence and reduce anxiety.

- **Change how you communicate** – Communicate at the child's level. Don't use ambiguous or non-literal language.

- **Recognise the behaviour that challenges** – In children with ASD, behaviour is unlikely to be a result of malice or naughtiness. All behaviour has a purpose; we need to take the time to be detectives and work out what is going on for a child.

- **Be consistent and realistic in your approach as a setting** – It is of key importance that everyone manages behaviour in the same way. You can use the behaviour plan outlined in (B3) to ensure a consistent approach.

# Making sense of behaviour

- **Plan transitions and changes to the routine** – Use a visual timetable (E5) and manage changes in the routine (E13).

- **Use appropriate rewards (this isn't bribery)** – Remember that most children with ASD are unlikely to do something just to make an adult happy. Use a child's individual motivators. Use the 'I am working for' chart in (B4).

- **Make your praise specific to encourage positive behaviours** – For example, Sari is sitting well on the carpet (whilst fiddling slightly with his shoe). If the adult says 'Good boy', how does Sari know which part of what he is doing that is 'good'? For a child who does not have a typical social understanding, he may feel that it is the fiddling with the shoe that is being labelled 'good'. Instead, use gestures and say 'Good sitting and good looking'. You may want to use visual supports to model the positive behaviours.

## Making sense of behaviour 1. The iceberg model

**B:1**

Use the iceberg model in your setting to help you separate out the behaviour (what you see on top) and what may be going on underneath in terms of a child's ASD.

Photocopy or draw out the model on a large sheet of paper (see the next page), and use it as a group to brainstorm. This is immensely helpful to do as a group to ensure shared understanding and consistency of approach.

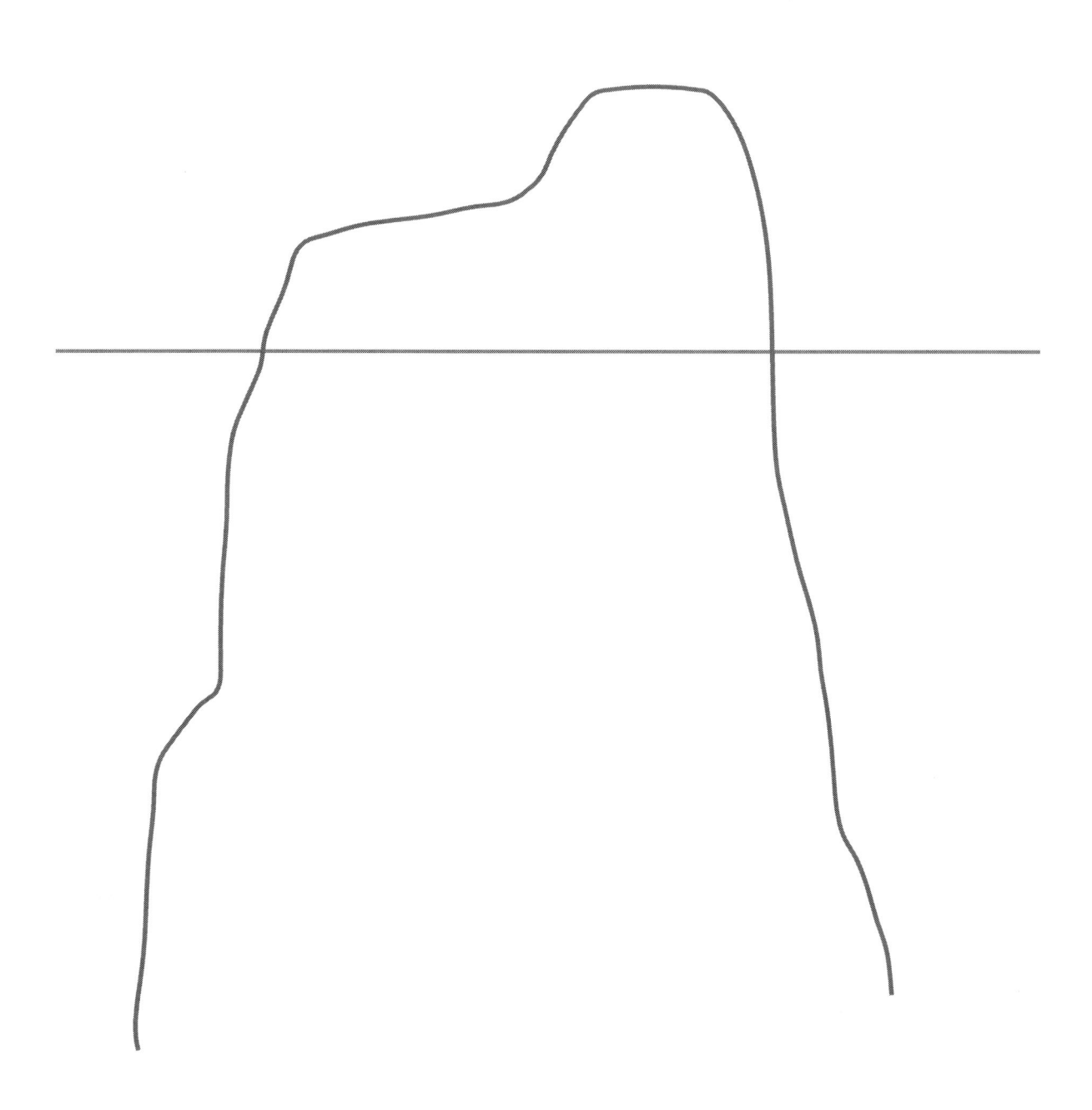

Copyright material from Jennifer Warwick (2020) *Supporting SLCN in Children with ASD in the Early Years*, Routledge

## Making sense of behaviour 2. ABC chart

**B:2**

As Dr McCarthy outlined, ABC charts are a good way of gathering information in detail, including what happened just before the behaviour occurred and what happened afterwards.

A stands for 'antecedent', which essentially means 'trigger' – that is, what triggered the behaviour?

The B stands for the 'behaviour' itself that you saw; it is helpful to describe the behaviour rather than label it.

The C stands for the 'consequence': what happened as a result of the behaviour. All of the elements are useful to consider. Keeping an ABC chart for at least a week helps build up a more detailed understanding of the factors that affect and keep the behaviour going.

| Date/time place | Antecedent | Behaviour | Consequence | Other observations |
|---|---|---|---|---|
|  |  |  |  |  |
|  |  |  |  |  |
|  |  |  |  |  |
|  |  |  |  |  |
|  |  |  |  |  |
|  |  |  |  |  |
|  |  |  |  |  |
|  |  |  |  |  |

## Making sense of behaviour 3.
## Pull it together – let's make a behaviour plan

**B:3**

A behaviour support plan can be a useful tool to pull together an action plan regarding how best to respond consistently to behaviour that a child may show. The plan outlines the behaviour you are looking to reduce and what you would like to see more of instead and how you plan to reach that. It is important in an education setting that all adults working with a child are aware of this, for example, reception staff, lunch time staff, and the playground supervisor.

| Behaviour support plan |  |
|---|---|
| **Child's name:**<br>**Date:**<br>**Written by:** |  |
| **Behaviour to reduce:**<br>(provide detailed description) |  |
| **Desired replacement behaviour:**<br>(what we would like to see instead – provide a detailed description) |  |
| **Strategies to encourage replacement behaviour:**<br>– Environment<br>– Visual supports<br>– Transitions<br>– Communication |  |
| **Potential triggers:** (antecedents) |  |
| **Preventative strategies:** |  |
| **Response strategy:** (what we do if the behaviour occurs) |  |

Copyright material from Jennifer Warwick (2020) *Supporting SLCN in Children with ASD in the Early Years*, Routledge

# Making sense of behaviour 4. 'I am working for'

We know that using visuals are a helpful way to enable children with ASD to learn. We can incorporate visuals as a reward to help motivate them to complete a task. The 'I am working for' board detailed as follows shows the child a motivating object or 'reinforcer' that they would like to achieve. To do this they need to receive three tokens or stars for completion. The stars could be for positive behaviour or completion of a task on a workstation. Once the child gets all the stars, he or she gets the motivating object. Remember that reinforcers are unique to the child; not everyone likes stickers or bubbles. Tailor the reward to the child's likes and motivations. You could use a visual choosing (C9) the child's favourite things for him or her to select the reward from.

**Photocopy the board and get started!**

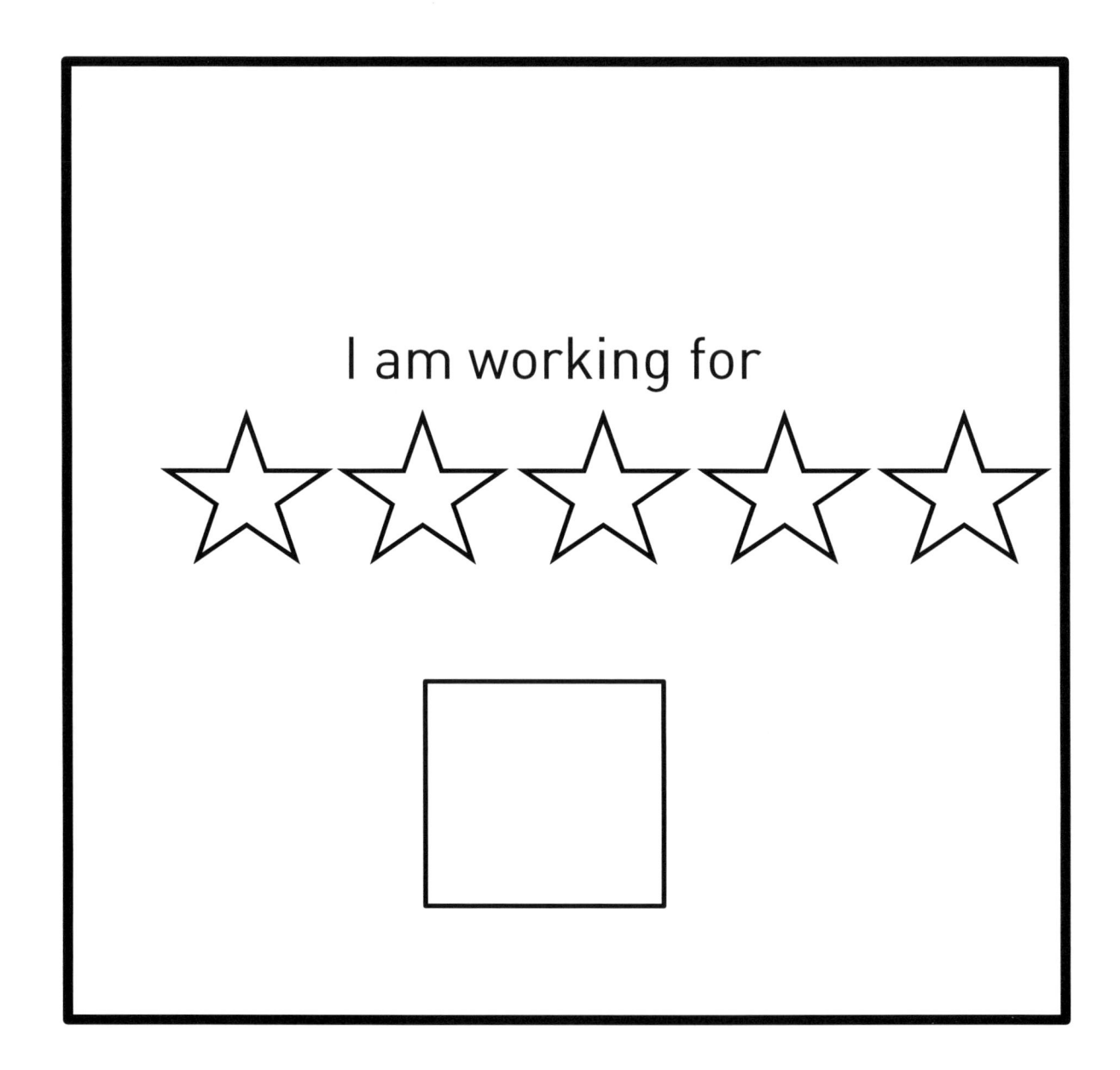

I am working for

☆☆☆☆☆

Copyright material from Jennifer Warwick (2020) *Supporting SLCN in Children with ASD in the Early Years*, Routledge

# Chapter Seven
# NEXT STEPS

This manual has provided you with relevant theory and practical activities to support SLCN in children with ASD within the early years environment. You can now confidently do the following:

- Apply your theoretical knowledge of ASD to 'get in the shoes' of a child with ASD.

- Use the Skills Profile and Information-Gathering Tool to gain insight into each individual child with ASD that you work with, remembering that just because children with ASD share a diagnosis, they may present very differently from each other.

- Understand how you can make changes to the environment to best support the SLCN of children with ASD.

- Adapt your style of communication to support children with ASD so that they can listen, understand, and communicate to the best of their abilities.

- Set up specific activities and use targeted strategies to support the SLCN of children with ASD.

- Support social communication and interaction in everyday activities by adapting what you are doing naturally.

- Facilitate play skills.

- Be a detective and try to work out why behaviours occur.

- Work collaboratively with families.

Before coming to an end, it is important to offer some closing reflections to support you in your next steps and moving forward:

- **Seek relevant support** – Find out what local services children can offer in your area. Be informed of relevant parent support groups and other local agencies that

# Next steps

you can link families into. The National Autistic Society runs a range of parent groups including local support groups (area dependent); the details are listed on their website, www.nas.org.

- **Develop your skills** – Access training wherever possible. ASD is an ever-evolving field, and there are always new and different approaches to be aware of. Find out if there are any ASD specials schools or resource bases in your area. Do they offer training or opportunities to observe?

- **Make timely referrals** – The provision of health and education services may be reduced depending on your local area. It is important to access SLT, OT, or education psychology if required. Ensure that you know the process to refer to local children's services in terms of information needed, referral forms, and so on.

- **Document everything** –Documenting meetings, goals, and outcomes is important in the process of applying for further support. Without this, it can be difficult to prove what you have put in place and what a child needs.

- **Give things time** – Strategies may not work straightaway. This is an important point and one that I often encounter in settings that have put excellent strategies in place and then feel despondent that they haven't seen immediate results. Allow six weeks before reviewing.

- **Involve parents** – Not only will this allow for consistency in application of strategies, but also parents know their children best. A collaborative approach is always good practise.

- **Reflect on the skills that you are developing** – You'll find them in yourself through this process and see the difference that you are making.

- **Acknowledge that it can be hard work** – Seek support and discussion from colleagues and relevant professionals to ensure that you are supported in your work. Although it can be hard work, it is extremely rewarding work supporting children to develop their ability to communicate and engage; you can make a real difference in many areas of their lives.

# APPENDICES

## Appendix One: Understanding ASD quiz

**A:1**

**Answers to the quiz on page 27**

**1   ASD is a neurological and developmental disorder that children are born with**

**TRUE** – *ASD is a neurological and developmental disorder that starts in early childhood and lasts throughout life. It is referred to as a spectrum as people may have a range of difficulties. All people with ASD will have difficulties in the areas of social communication and interaction and restricted and repetitive behaviours.*

**2   People with ASD experience the world differently**

**TRUE** – *We know that this is true from the testimonies of people with ASD. Sensory difficulties combined with the other core difficulties associated with ASD mean that the world can be different for people with ASD. This is important to bear in mind in your work with young children.*

**3   Children can grow out of ASD**

**FALSE** – *Children with ASD grow up to be adults with ASD. The profile of needs will change over time, and undoubtedly early intervention and therapy can help but it is not possible to grow out of ASD.*

**4   Once children can talk their ASD almost disappears**

**FALSE** – *This is a common misconception. Talking is a helpful skill to learn, but verbal children with ASD continue to have social interaction and communication difficulties.*

**5   There are more boys with ASD than girls**

**TRUE** – *Current figures currently cite a four-to-one ratio of boys to girls; however, we know that many girls are missed or misdiagnosed. Increasing research shows that girls with ASD present differently from boys.*

**6   How many people in the UK have ASD?**
   One in 1000
   One in 100
   One in 10 000

*Current rates of diagnosis cite one in 100.*

## Appendices

**7   Parents of children with ASD are to blame for their child's difficulties**

**FALSE** – *This is completely false. ASD was originally blamed on 'refrigerator mothers', but this is an outdated theory.*

**8   What two areas does a person need to have difficulties in to get a diagnosis of ASD?**

*To get a diagnosis of ASD, a person needs to show difficulties in the areas of social communication and interaction and restricted and repetitive behaviours.*

**9   Vaccines cause ASD**

*This is completely false but is a damaging myth relating to ASD. In 1998 a study based on only twelve children suggested that ASD was related to the MMR vaccine. This study has been disproven and discredited and the author struck off the UK medical register.*

**10   All people with ASD have sensory processing difficulties**

**FALSE** –*Not everyone with a diagnosis of ASD will have sensory processing difficulties. We do know that the impact of sensory difficulties can be significant.*

## Appendix Two: Strategy planning

**A:2**

Throughout this manual we mention the importance of consistency.

Less is more! Rather than choosing a wide number of goals for a child and everyone implementing them in a disjointed manner, it is much more effective for staff working with a child to work on one strategy at a time and implementing it consistently.

The strategy planner on the next page can be used as a template to plan what strategies will be used and the impact that these will have.

| | |
|---|---|
| **Child's name:**<br>**Date:** | |
| **Date of planning:** | |
| **Strategy/activity to be introduced:**<br>*Outline as much as possible what you will be doing with the child.* | |
| **How will this help:**<br>*Be specific; try to imagine what difference this will make.* | |
| **What will be different for the child:**<br>*Be specific; this will help motivate you. It also provides a basis for thinking about the progress that he or she is going to make.* | |
| **How to implement the strategy:**<br>*What actions are needed to ensure consistency? It can be useful to agree about these with parents and all those who spend time with a child.* | |

Copyright material from Jennifer Warwick (2020) *Supporting SLCN in Children with ASD in the Early Years*, Routledge

## Appendix Three: Let's create planning sheet

A:3

- ✓ **What is the activity:**
- ✓ **What do I need:**
- ✓ **What do I want 'the child to do':**
- ✓ **What strategies can I use to support this:**
- ✓ **How can I start the activity:**
- ✓ **How can I finish the activity:**

| Child's name: Date: | |
|---|---|
| Activity: | |
| Materials needed: | |
| Goals (for child): *This is the key bit: what we want the child to be doing differently* | |
| Strategies to support: | |
| How can I start the activity: | |
| How can I finish the activity: | |
| Other comments: | |

Copyright material from Jennifer Warwick (2020) *Supporting SLCN in Children with ASD in the Early Years*, Routledge

Appendices

## Appendix Four: Communication profile

**A:4**

Using a profile like that on the next page is a useful way to easily share information about a child so that all staff and visitors to the setting are aware of an individual child's strengths and needs.

| My name is . . . |
| Please read this to learn more about me and how I communicate. |

| About me: | How I communicate: |
|---|---|
| | |

| I am working on: | You can help me by: |
|---|---|
| | |

If you have any questions, please talk to my key worker.

Appendices

## Appendix Five: Interaction planner

A:5

Breaking an interaction down to each part can seem like a lot to do! Stick with it, as once you have done it a few times, you will cue into thinking how you can use these strategies to support the children with ASD who you are working with.

Use the template on the next page to plan an interaction.

| **Child's name:**<br>**Date:**<br>**Activity:** | |
|---|---|
| How will I start the game (same way every time): | |
| What gestures/actions shall I use: | |
| Where will I pause: | |
| Goals (for child): | |
| Strategies to use: | |
| How will I keep it fun: | |
| How will I end the game: | |

# Appendices

See the sample interaction planner completed for Adam (Chapter One).

Adam's interaction planner

| **Child's name: Adam**<br>**Date: 16.9.2019**<br>**Activity: Ring a Round a Roses (a joint game with an adult and two peers)** | |
|---|---|
| How will I start the game (same way every time): | • Show Adam the song symbol<br>• Put my hands out in a consistent gesture<br>• Say, 'Let's play Ring a Round' |
| What gestures/actions shall I use: | • Natural gesture and signs to accompany speech<br>• Pointing |
| Where will I pause: | • At high points in the game, wait expectantly for Adam to fill in the gaps |
| Goals (for child): | • For Adam to have a positive social experience with peers<br>• For Adam to request more of an interaction<br>• For Adam to engage in a structured game with peers |
| Strategies to use: | • Pausing<br>• Making a chance to communicate |
| How will I keep it fun: | Through motivating facial expressions and sounds |
| How will I end the game: | Give one-minute warning and say, 'Singing has finished'; show Adam what is next on first/then board |

Printed in Great Britain
by Amazon